CONTENTS

About This Booklet 1

Eating Well During Cancer Treatment 2
   What Kinds of Food Do I Need? 2
   Figure 1. Eat a Variety of Foods Each Day 4
   Sample Menu for Good Nutrition 5
   Can Good Nutrition Treat Cancer? 6

Managing Eating Problems During Treatment 7
   Figure 2. How Cancer Treatments Can Affect Eating 8
   Coping With Side Effects 9
      Loss of Appetite 9
      Sore Mouth or Throat 10
      Changed Sense of Taste or Smell 12
      Dry Mouth 13
      Nausea 14
      Vomiting 15
      Diarrhea 16
      Constipation 18
      Weight Gain 19
      Tooth Decay 19
      Lactose Intolerance 20
   Saving Time and Energy 20
      Table 1. Snacks 22
   Improving Your Nutrition 23
      Table 2. How To Increase Protein 24
      Table 3. How To Increase Calories 26

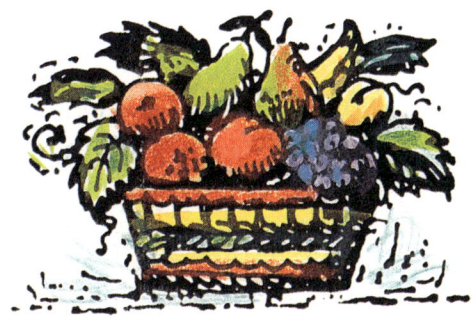

Special Diets for Special Needs 29
    Clear-Liquid Diet 30
    Full-Liquid Diet 32
    Soft-Diet 34
    Fiber-Restricted Diet 37
    Low-Lactose Diet 41
    Commercial Products To Improve Nutrition 45

Resources 46
Glossary 47
Recipes for Better Nutrition During Cancer Treatment 50
Recipe Index 93

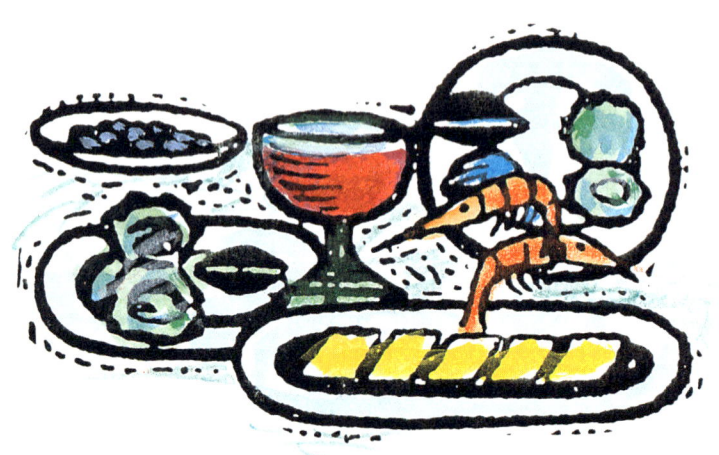

ABOUT THIS BOOKLET

Your diet is an important part of your treatment for cancer. Eating the right kinds of foods during your treatment can help you feel better and stay stronger.

The National Cancer Institute (NCI) has prepared this booklet to help you learn more about your diet needs and how to manage eating problems. Eating well is extra important when your body is fighting disease.

This booklet is mainly for patients who are still receiving cancer treatment. However, it also may be useful after you finish treatment. Pick it up any time you find that eating well is a challenge.

You may not want to read all of this booklet at one sitting. Flip through it to see which sections are useful to you now. Save it so that you can refer to other sections as needed.

Your registered dietitian, doctor, and nurse are your best sources of information about your diet. The information in this booklet will add to their advice. Feel free to ask them for help and to talk with them about changes in your diet. Ask them to explain or repeat anything that is not clear.

In the "Resources" section of this booklet, which begins on page 46, you will find information about other free NCI publications about cancer, its treatment, and coping with the illness. We also have listed the American Cancer Society (ACS) and the NCI-supported Cancer Information Service (CIS) (1-800-4-CANCER).

The CIS provides information about cancer, cancer treatment, research studies, and living with cancer to patients, their families, health professionals, and the public.

The "Glossary," on pages 47-49, lists and defines words that relate to diet, nutrition, and other aspects of cancer care. Words appearing in **bold** throughout this booklet are defined in the Glossary. A section on "Recipes for Better Nutrition During Cancer Treatment," which begins on page 50, was written to help you solve some of the nutritional problems you may have during your treatment. Many of these recipes are from patients and family members who wanted to share their tips for better eating.

EATING WELL DURING CANCER TREATMENT

A nutritious **diet** is always vital for your body to work at its best. Good **nutrition** is even more important for people with cancer. Why?

- Patients who eat well during their treatment are able to cope better with the side effects of treatment. Patients who eat well may be able to handle a higher dose of certain treatments.
- A healthy diet can help keep up your strength, prevent body tissues from breaking down, and rebuild tissues that cancer treatment may harm.
- When you are unable to eat enough food or the right kind of food, your body uses stored **nutrients** as a source of energy. As a result, your natural defenses are weaker and your body cannot fight **infection** as well. Yet, this defense system is especially important to you now, because cancer patients are often at risk of getting an infection.

What Kinds of Food Do I Need?

A good rule to follow is to eat a variety of different foods every day. No one food or group of foods contains all of the nutrients you need. A diet to keep your body strong will include daily servings from these food groups:

Fruits and Vegetables: Raw or cooked vegetables, fruits, and fruit juices provide certain **vitamins** (such as A and C) and **minerals** the body needs.

Protein Foods: **Protein** helps your body heal itself and fight infection. Meat, fish, poultry, eggs, milk, yogurt, and cheese give you protein as well as many vitamins and minerals.

Grains: Grains, such as bread, pasta, rice, and cereals, provide a variety of **carbohydrates** and B vitamins. Carbohydrates provide a good source of energy, which the body needs to function well.

Dairy Foods: Milk and other dairy products provide protein and many vitamins and are the best source of calcium.

To help Americans learn how to choose a healthy diet, the U.S. Department of Agriculture and the U.S. Department of Health and Human Services designed a Food Guide Pyramid. The Food Guide Pyramid gives the amounts and types of foods most Americans should try to eat each day. It emphasizes five food groups — Bread, Fruit, Vegetable, Milk, and Meat — and focuses on reducing the amount of fat in the diet. The chart on page 4, "Eat a Variety of Foods Each Day," gives more details about the guidelines in the Pyramid. The sample menu on page 5 shows one way you can follow the Food Pyramid guidelines.

Keep in mind that the Food Pyramid may not meet the needs of individuals with special diet needs, such as cancer patients. In fact, *the best foods for you right now may be very different from those in the Food Pyramid, depending on the type of treatment you are receiving or how you feel.* You probably will need more calories and more high-protein foods, such as meats and dairy products. You may need to cut back on high-fiber foods for a while, such as vegetables, fruits, cereals, and whole grains, if your treatment causes diarrhea. Your doctor, nurse, or **registered dietitian** also may suggest that you add commercial nutrition supplements to your diet to make sure you get enough protein, **calories**, and other nutrients during treatment. (See the section, "Commercial Products To Improve Nutrition," on page 45.)

Pay attention to your body. If nausea makes certain foods unappealing, then eat more of the foods you find easier to handle. For example, if you get nauseous from eating fruits but can eat protein foods, eat more protein foods and less fruit.

Sometimes changing the form of a food will make it more appetizing and help you eat better. You might try mixing canned fruit into a milkshake if eating whole, fresh fruits is a problem.

It is important to keep trying new things. Anything you eat will be a plus in helping you get enough calories

Figure 1. EAT A VARIETY OF FOODS EACH DAY

Food Group	Suggested Daily Servings	What Counts As a Serving?
Breads, Cereals, Rice, Pasta, and Other Grain Products Whole-grain enriched	6-11 servings from entire group (include several servings of whole-grain products daily)	■ 1 slice of bread ■ 1/2 hamburger bun or English muffin ■ 1 small roll, biscuit, or muffin ■ 3 to 4 small or 2 large crackers ■ 1/2 cup cooked cereal, rice, or pasta ■ 1 oz. of ready-to-eat breakfast cereals
Fruits Citrus, melon, berries, other fruits	2-3 servings from entire group	■ 1 medium apple, banana, peach, pear, etc. ■ 1 grapefruit half ■ 1 melon wedge ■ 3/4 cup of juice ■ 1/2 cup of berries ■ 1/2 cup chopped, cooked, or canned fruit ■ 1/4 cup dried fruit
Vegetables Dark-green leafy Deep-yellow Legumes (e.g., navy, pinto, and kidney beans; chickpeas) Starchy Other vegetables	3-5 servings from entire group (include all types regularly); use dark-green leafy vegetables and legumes several times a week	■ 3/4 cup of vegetable juice ■ 1 cup of leafy raw vegetables (e.g., spinach) ■ 1/2 cup non-leafy vegetables (cooked or chopped raw)
Meat, Poultry, Fish, Dry Beans, Eggs, and Nuts	2-3 servings from entire group	Amounts should total 5 to 7 oz. of cooked lean meat, poultry, or fish each day. Count 1 egg; 1/2 cup cooked dried beans, peas, or seeds; and 2 tbsp. peanut butter as 1 oz. of meat

and maintain your weight. This booklet describes some of the special diets that cancer patients may need to follow. (See "Special Diets for Special Needs," on page 29.) It also gives ideas and recipes that worked for other cancer patients when they had to change their diet or when they didn't feel like eating.

Your doctor, nurse, and registered dietitian will let you know which diet is best for you. Be sure to talk with them if you have any questions.

<td colspan="3" align="center">***Figure 1.* (continued)**</td>
Food Group	**Suggested Daily Servings**	**What Counts As a Serving?**
Milk, Yogurt, and Cheese	2-3 servings from entire group (3 servings for teenagers, adults under 25, and women who are pregnant or breast-feeding; 4 servings for teens who are pregnant or breastfeeding)	■ 1 cup of milk ■ 8 oz. of yogurt ■ 1 1/2 oz. of natural cheese ■ 2 oz. of processed cheese
Fats, Oils, Sweets, and Alcoholic Beverages	Use sparingly. Use unsaturated vegetable oils and margarines that list a liquid vegetable oil as the first ingredient on the label. If you drink alcoholic beverages, do so in moderation.	■ 1 tbsp. mayonnaise or dressing ■ 1 tsp. butter or margarine ■ 2 tbsp. sour cream or cream cheese ■ 1 tsp. sugar, jam, or jelly ■ 1 12-oz. soda ■ 1/2 cup fruit sorbet or gelatin ■ 1 oz. candy ■ 1 tsp. salt ■ 1 oz. (about 14) potato chips ■ 1 tbsp. catsup, mustard, steak sauce, or soy sauce
Source: USDA Food Guide Pyramid		

The following sample menu supplies the minimum number of servings from each food group. If you need to include extra calories or protein in your diet, add more servings and include snacks, appetizers, desserts, and drinks from the lists on pages 22 and 24-27.

Sample Food Menu for Good Nutrition

Breakfast
1/2 cup cooked cereal
1/2 cup milk
1/2 cup fruit or fruit juice
Beverage (coffee, tea, water)
Sugar

Snack
1/4 cup granola
1/2 cup low-fat yogurt

Lunch
Sandwich:
    2 slices whole-grain bread
    2-3 oz. lean meat, fish, or poultry
    1 tsp. mayonnaise
    lettuce, tomato slices
1 piece fruit
Beverage

Snack
1/2 cup raw vegetables with
    1 tbsp. salad dressing

Dinner
2-3 oz. lean meat, fish,
    or poultry
1 cup steamed vegetables
1/2 cup grain product
    (e.g., pasta or brown rice)
1 tsp. margarine or butter
1 cup milk
Beverage

Snack
4 whole wheat crackers
1 tbsp. jelly
Beverage

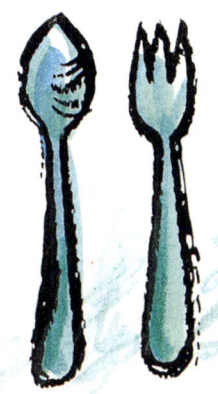

Can Good Nutrition Treat Cancer?

Doctors know that patients who eat well during cancer treatment are better able to cope with side effects caused by treatment. *However, there is no evidence that any kind of diet or food can either cure cancer or stop it from coming back.* In fact, some diets may be harmful, especially those that don't include a variety of foods. There is also no evidence that dietary supplements, such as vitamin or mineral pills, can cure cancer or stop it from coming back.

The NCI strongly urges you to eat nutritious foods and follow the treatment program prescribed by a doctor who uses accepted and proven methods or treatments. People who depend upon unconventional treatments may lose valuable treatment time and reduce their chances of controlling cancer and getting well.

The NCI also recommends that you ask your doctor, nurse, or registered dietitian before taking any vitamins or mineral supplements. Too much of some vitamins or minerals can be just as dangerous as too little. Large doses of some vitamins may even stop your cancer treatment from working the way it should. To avoid problems, don't take these products on your own. Follow your doctor's directions for safe results.

Managing Eating Problems During Treatment

All the methods of treating cancer—surgery, **radiation therapy**, **chemotherapy**, and **biological therapy (immunotherapy)**—are very powerful. Although treatments target the cancer cells in your body, they sometimes can damage normal, healthy cells at the same time. This may produce unpleasant side effects that cause eating problems. (See Figure 2.)

Side effects of cancer treatment vary from patient to patient. The part of the body being treated, length of treatment, and the dose of treatment also affect whether side effects will occur. Ask your doctor about how your treatment may affect you.

The good news is that only about one-third of cancer patients have side effects during treatment, and most side effects go away when treatment ends. Your doctor will try to plan a treatment that keeps side effects down.

Cancer treatment also may affect your eating in another way. When some people are upset, worried, or afraid, they may have eating problems. Losing your appetite and nausea are two normal responses to feeling nervous or fearful. Such problems should last only a short time.

While you are in the hospital, members of the food or nutrition service, including a registered dietitian, can help you plan your diet. They also can help you solve your physical or emotional eating problems. Feel free to talk to them if problems arise during your recovery as well. Ask them what has worked for their other patients.

Don't be afraid to give food a chance. Not everyone has problems with eating during cancer treatment. Even those who have eating problems have days when eating is a pleasure.

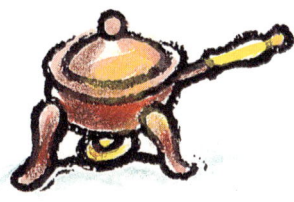

Figure 2. HOW CANCER TREATMENTS CAN AFFECT EATING

Cancer Treatment	How It Can Affect Eating	What Sometimes Happens: Side Effects
Surgery	Increases the need for good nutrition because it puts stress on the body. May slow digestion. May lessen the ability of the mouth, throat, and stomach to work properly. Also may make the mouth, throat, and stomach sore.	Before surgery, a high-protein, high-calorie diet may be prescribed if a patient is underweight or weak. After surgery, some patients may not resume normal eating at first. They may receive nutrients: ■ Through a needle in their vein (**IV or intravenous feeding**). ■ Through a tube in their nose or stomach. ■ By drinking clear liquids (see pages 30-31). ■ By following a full-liquid diet (see pages 32-33).
Radiation Therapy	As it damages cancer cells, it also may damage healthy cells and healthy parts of the body.	Treatment of head, neck, or chest may cause: ■ Dry mouth. ■ Sore mouth. ■ Sore throat. ■ Difficulty swallowing (dysphagia). ■ Change in taste of food. ■ Dental problems. Treatment of stomach may cause: ■ Nausea. ■ Vomiting. ■ Diarrhea.
Chemotherapy	As it destroys cancer cells, it also may harm parts of the body needed for eating.	■ Nausea and vomiting. ■ Loss of appetite. ■ Diarrhea. ■ Constipation. ■ Sore mouth or throat. ■ Weight gain. ■ Change in taste of food.
Biological Therapy (Immunotherapy)	Not known.	■ Nausea and vomiting. ■ Diarrhea. ■ Sore mouth. ■ Severe weight loss (anorexia). ■ Dry mouth. ■ Change in taste of food.

Coping With Side Effects

This section offers practical hints for coping with treatment side effects that may affect your eating.

These suggestions have helped other patients manage eating problems that can be frustrating to handle. Try all the ideas to find what works best for you. Share your needs and concerns with your family and friends, particularly those who prepare meals for you. Let them know that you appreciate their support as you work to take control of eating problems.

Loss of Appetite

Loss of appetite or poor appetite is one of the most common problems that occurs with cancer and its treatment. Many things affect appetite, including feeling sick (having nausea, vomiting) and being upset or depressed about having cancer. A person who has these feelings, whether physical or emotional, may not be interested in eating.

You may find the following suggestions helpful in making mealtimes more relaxed so that you will feel more like eating.

- Stay calm, especially at mealtimes. Don't hurry your meals.
- Involve yourself in as many normal activities as possible. But, if you feel uneasy and do not want to take part, don't force yourself.
- Try changing the time, place, and surroundings of meals. A candlelight dinner can make mealtime more appealing. Set a colorful table. Listen to soft music while eating. Eat with others or watch your favorite TV program while you eat.

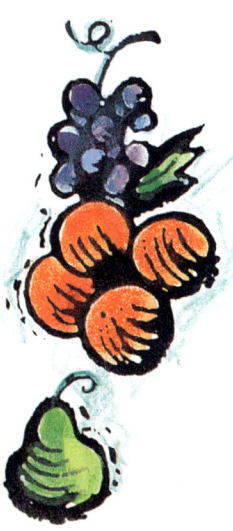

- Eat whenever you are hungry. You do not need to eat just three main meals a day. Several small meals throughout the day may be even better.
- Add variety to your menu. Try some of the recipes in the "Recipes for Better Nutrition During Cancer Treatment" section of this book.
- Eat food often during the day, even at bedtime. Have healthy snacks handy. Taking just a few bites of the right foods or sips of the right liquids every hour or so can help you get more protein and calories. You can find ideas for preparing snacks on page 22.

Sore Mouth or Throat

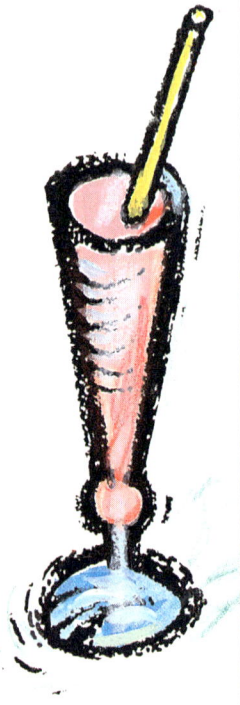

Mouth sores, tender gums, and a sore throat or esophagus often result from radiation therapy, anti-cancer drugs, and infection. If you have a sore mouth or gums, see your doctor to be sure the soreness is a treatment side effect and not an unrelated dental problem. The doctor may be able to give you medicine that will control mouth and throat pain. Your dentist also can give you tips for care of your mouth.

Certain foods will irritate an already tender mouth and make chewing and swallowing difficult. By carefully choosing the foods you eat and by taking good care of your mouth, you can usually make eating easier. Here are some suggestions that may help:

- Try soft foods that are easy to chew and swallow, such as:
  —Milkshakes.
  —Bananas, applesauce, and other soft fruits.
  —Peach, pear, and apricot nectars.
  —Watermelon.
  —Cottage cheese.
  —Mashed potatoes, macaroni and cheese.
  —Custards, puddings, and gelatin.

- —Scrambled eggs.
- —Oatmeal or other cooked cereals.
- —Pureed or mashed vegetables such as peas and carrots.
- —Pureed meats.
- —Liquids.

- Avoid foods that can irritate your mouth, such as:
  - —Citrus fruit or juice such as oranges, grapefruits, tangerines.
  - —Spicy or salty foods.
  - —Rough, coarse, or dry foods such as raw vegetables, granola, toast, crackers.
- Cook foods until they are soft and tender.
- Cut foods into small pieces.
- Mix food with butter, thin gravies, and sauces to make it easier to swallow.
- Use a blender or food processor to puree your food.
- Use a straw to drink liquids.
- Try foods cold or at room temperature. Hot and warm foods can irritate a tender mouth and throat.
- If swallowing is hard, tilting your head back or moving it forward may help.
- If heartburn is a problem, try sitting up or standing for about an hour after eating.
- If your teeth and gums are sore, your dentist may be able to recommend a special product for cleaning your teeth.
- Rinse your mouth with water often to remove food and bacteria and to promote healing.
- Ask your doctor about anesthetic lozenges and sprays that can numb the mouth and throat long enough for you to eat meals.

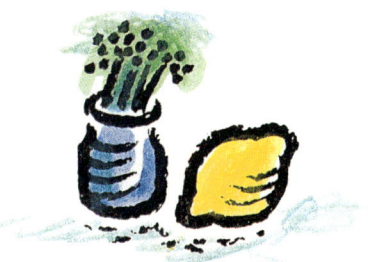

Changed Sense of Taste or Smell

Your sense of taste or smell may change during your illness or treatment. A condition called mouth blindness or taste blindness may give foods a bitter or metallic taste, especially meat or other high-protein foods. Many foods will have less taste. Chemotherapy, radiation therapy, or the cancer itself may cause these problems. Dental problems also can change the way foods taste. For most people, changes in taste and smell go away when their treatment is finished.

There is no "foolproof" way to improve the flavor or smell of food because each person is affected differently by illness and treatments. However, the tips given below should help make your food taste better. *(If you also have a sore mouth, sore gums, or a sore throat, talk to your doctor or registered dietitian. They can suggest ways to improve the taste of your food without hurting the sore areas.)*

- Choose and prepare foods that look and smell good to you.
- If red meat (such as beef) tastes or smells strange, use chicken, turkey, eggs, dairy products, or fish that doesn't have a strong smell instead.
- Help the flavor of meat, chicken, or fish by marinating it in sweet fruit juices, sweet wine, Italian dressing, or sweet-and-sour sauce.
- Try using small amounts of flavorful seasonings such as basil, oregano, or rosemary.
- Try tart foods such as oranges or lemonade that may have more taste. A tart lemon custard might taste good and will also provide needed protein and calories. *(Do not try this if you have a sore mouth or throat.)*
- Serve foods at room temperature.
- Try using bacon, ham, or onion to add flavor to vegetables.

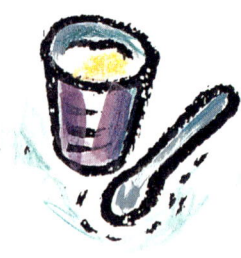

- Stop eating foods that cause an unpleasant taste.
- Visit your dentist to rule out dental problems that may affect the taste or smell of food.
- Ask your dentist about special mouthwashes and good mouth care.

Dry Mouth

Chemotherapy and radiation therapy in the head or neck area can reduce the flow of saliva and often cause dry mouth. When this happens, foods are harder to chew and swallow. Dry mouth also can change the way foods taste. The suggestions below may be helpful in dealing with dry mouth. Also try some of the ideas for dealing with a sore mouth or throat, which can make foods easier to swallow.

- Try very sweet or tart foods and beverages such as lemonade; these foods may help your mouth produce more saliva. *(Do not try this if you also have a tender mouth or sore throat.)*
- Suck on sugar-free, hard candy or popsicles or chew sugar-free gum. These can help produce more saliva.
- Use soft and pureed foods, which may be easier to swallow.
- Keep your lips moist with lip salves.
- Eat foods with sauces, gravies, and salad dressings to make them moist and easier to swallow.
- Have a sip of water every few minutes to help you swallow and talk more easily.
- If your dry mouth problem is severe, ask your doctor or dentist about products that coat and protect your mouth and throat.

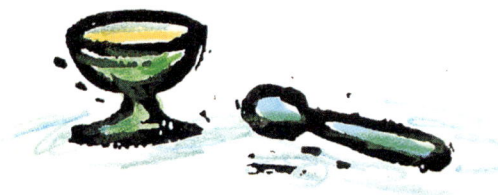

Nausea

Nausea, with or without vomiting, is a common side effect of surgery, chemotherapy, radiation therapy, and biological therapy. The disease itself, or other conditions unrelated to your cancer or treatment, also may cause nausea.

Whatever the cause, nausea can keep you from getting enough food and needed nutrients. Here are some ideas that may be helpful:

- Ask your doctor about medicine to help control nausea and vomiting. These drugs are called **antiemetics**.
- Try these foods:
  - Toast and crackers.
  - Yogurt.
  - Sherbet.
  - Pretzels.
  - Angel food cake.
  - Oatmeal.
  - Skinned chicken (baked or broiled, not fried).
  - Fruits and vegetables that are soft or bland, such as canned peaches.
  - Clear liquids, sipped slowly.
  - Ice chips.
- Avoid these foods:
  - Fatty, greasy, or fried.
  - Very sweet, such as candy, cookies, or cake.
  - Spicy or hot.
  - With strong odors.
- Eat small amounts often and slowly.
- Avoid eating in a room that's stuffy, too warm, or has cooking odors that might disagree with you.
- Drink fewer liquids with meals. Drinking liquids can cause a full, bloated feeling.
- Drink or sip liquids throughout the day, *except* at mealtimes. Using a straw may help.
- Drink beverages cool or chilled. Try freezing favorite beverages in ice cube trays.

- Eat foods at room temperature or cooler; hot foods may add to nausea.
- Don't force yourself to eat favorite foods when you feel nauseated. This may cause a permanent dislike of those foods.
- Rest after meals, because activity may slow digestion. It's best to rest sitting up for about an hour after meals.
- If nausea is a problem in the morning, try eating dry toast or crackers before getting up.
- Wear loose-fitting clothes.
- Avoid eating for 1 to 2 hours before treatment if nausea occurs during radiation therapy or chemotherapy.
- Try to keep track of when your nausea occurs and what causes it (specific foods, events, surroundings). If possible, make appropriate changes in your diet or schedule. Share the information with your doctor or nurse.

Vomiting

Vomiting may follow nausea and may be brought on by treatment, food odors, gas in the stomach or bowel, or motion. In some people, certain surroundings, such as the hospital, may cause vomiting.

If vomiting is severe or lasts for more than a few days, contact your doctor.

Very often, if you can control nausea, you can prevent vomiting. At times, though, you may not be able to prevent either nausea or vomiting. You may find some relief by using relaxation exercises or meditation. These usually involve deep rhythmic breathing and quiet concentration and can be done almost anywhere. If vomiting occurs, try these hints to prevent further episodes.

- Ask your doctor about medicine to control nausea and vomiting (antiemetics).

- Do not drink or eat until you have the vomiting under control.
- Once you have controlled vomiting, try small amounts of clear liquids. (See pages 30-31.) Begin with 1 teaspoonful every 10 minutes, gradually increase the amount to 1 tablespoonful every 20 minutes, and finally, try 2 tablespoonfuls every 30 minutes.
- When you are able to keep down clear liquids, try a full-liquid diet. (See pages 32-33.) Continue taking small amounts as often as you can keep them down. If you feel okay on a full-liquid diet, gradually work up to your regular diet. If you have a hard time digesting milk, you may want to try a soft diet instead of a full-liquid diet. When you feel okay on the soft diet, gradually add more foods to return to your regular diet. (You can find information about these and other diets under "Special Diets for Special Needs," on page 29.)

Diarrhea

Diarrhea may have several causes, including chemotherapy, radiation therapy to the abdomen, infection, food sensitivity, and emotional upset.

Long-term or severe diarrhea may cause other problems. During diarrhea, food passes quickly through the bowel before the body absorbs enough vitamins, minerals, and water. This may cause **dehydration** and increase the risk of infection. Contact your doctor if the diarrhea is severe or lasts for more than a couple of days. Here are some ideas for coping with diarrhea:

- Drink plenty of liquids during the day. Drinking fluids is important because your body may not get enough water when you have diarrhea.
- Eat small amounts of food throughout the day instead of three large meals.

- Eat plenty of foods and liquids that contain **sodium** (salt) and **potassium**. These minerals are often lost during diarrhea. Good liquid choices include bouillon or fat-free broth. Foods high in potassium that don't cause diarrhea include bananas, peach and apricot nectar, and boiled or mashed potatoes.
- Try these nutritious low-fiber foods:
  — Yogurt.
  — Rice or noodles.
  — Grape juice.
  — Farina or cream of wheat.
  — Eggs (cooked until the whites are solid, not fried).
  — Ripe bananas.
  — Smooth peanut butter.
  — White bread.
  — Skinned chicken or turkey, lean beef, or fish (boiled or baked, not fried).
  — Cottage cheese, cream cheese.
- Eliminate foods such as:
  — Greasy, fatty, or fried foods.
  — Raw vegetables and fruits.
  — High-fiber vegetables such as broccoli, corn, beans, cabbage, peas, and cauliflower.
  — Strong spices, such as hot pepper, curry, and Cajun spice mix.
- Drink liquids that are at room temperature.
- Avoid very hot or very cold foods and beverages.
- Limit foods and beverages that contain caffeine, such as coffee, strong tea, some sodas, and chocolate.
- Be careful when using milk and milk products because diarrhea may be caused by **lactose intolerance**. (If you think you have this problem, see "Low-Lactose Diet," on pages 42 to 43.) Ask your doctor or registered dietitian for advice.

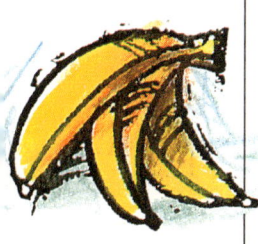

17

- After sudden, short-term attacks of diarrhea (acute diarrhea), try a clear-liquid diet during the first 12 to 14 hours. This lets the bowel rest while replacing the important body fluids lost during diarrhea. (Guidelines for a Clear-Liquid Diet appear on pages 30-31.)

Constipation

Some anticancer drugs and other drugs, such as pain medicines, may cause constipation. This problem also may occur if your diet lacks enough fluid or bulk or if you have been bedridden.

Here are some suggestions to prevent and treat constipation:

- Drink plenty of liquids—at least eight 8-ounce glasses every day. This will help to keep your stools soft.
- Take a hot drink about one-half hour before your usual time for a bowel movement.
- Eat high-fiber foods, such as whole-grain breads, cereals, and pastas; fresh fruits and vegetables; dried beans and peas; and whole-grain products such as barley or brown rice. Eat the skin on fruits and potatoes.
- Get some exercise, such as walking, every day. Talk to your doctor or a physical therapist about the amount and type of exercise that is right for you.
- Add unprocessed wheat bran to foods such as cereals, casseroles, and homemade breads.

If these suggestions don't work, ask your doctor about medicine to ease constipation. *Be sure to check with your doctor before taking any laxatives or stool softeners.*

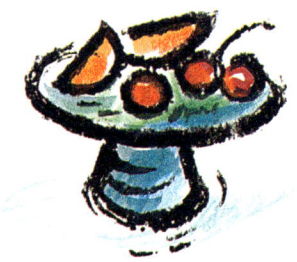

Weight Gain

Sometimes patients gain excess weight during treatment without eating extra calories. For example, certain anticancer drugs, such as prednisone, can cause the body to hold on to fluid causing weight gain; this condition is known as **edema**. The extra weight is in the form of water and does not mean you are eating too much.

It is important not to go on a diet if you notice weight gain. Instead, tell your doctor so you can find out what may be causing this change. If anticancer drugs are causing your body to retain water, your doctor may ask you to speak with a registered dietitian. The registered dietitian can teach you how to limit the amount of salt you eat, which is important because salt causes your body to hold extra water. Drugs called **diuretics** also may be prescribed to get rid of extra fluid.

Tooth Decay

Cancer and cancer treatment can cause tooth decay and other problems for your teeth and gums. Changes in eating habits also may add to the problem. If you eat often or eat a lot of sweets, you may need to brush your teeth more often. Brushing after each meal or snack is a good idea.

Here are some ideas for preventing dental problems:

- Be sure to see your dentist regularly. Patients who are receiving treatment that affects the mouth (e.g., radiation to the head and neck) may need to see the dentist more often than usual.
- Use a soft toothbrush. Ask your doctor, nurse, or dentist to suggest a special kind of toothbrush and/or toothpaste if your gums are very sensitive.
- Rinse your mouth with warm water when your gums and mouth are sore.
- If you are not having trouble with poor appetite or weight loss, limit the amount of sugar in your diet.
- Avoid eating foods that stick to the teeth, such as caramels or chewy candy bars.

Lactose Intolerance

Lactose intolerance means that your body can't digest or absorb the milk sugar called lactose. Milk, other dairy products, and foods to which milk has been added contain lactose.

Lactose intolerance may occur after treatment with some antibiotics or with radiation to the stomach or any treatment that affects the digestive tract. The part of your intestines that breaks down lactose may not work properly during treatment. For some people the symptoms of lactose intolerance (gas, cramping, diarrhea) disappear a few weeks or months after the treatments end or when the intestine heals. For others a permanent change in eating habits may be needed.

If you have this problem, your doctor may advise you to follow a diet that is low in foods that contain lactose. (See "Low-Lactose Diet" on pages 42-43.) If milk had been a main source of protein in your diet, it will be important to get enough protein from other foods. Products such as soybean formulas and aged cheeses are good sources of protein and other nutrients. You also may want to try low-lactose milk or use liquid drops or caplets that help break down the lactose in milk and other dairy products. The recipes beginning on page 50 can give you ideas for preparing low-lactose dishes.

Saving Time and Energy

Your body needs both rest and nourishment during and after treatment for cancer. If you are usually the cook, here are some suggestions for saving time and energy in preparing meals.

- Let someone else do the cooking when possible.
- If you know that your recovery time from treatment or surgery is going to be longer than 1 or 2 days, prepare a helper list. Decide who can

help you shop, cook, set the table, and clean up. Write it down, discuss it, and post it where it can easily be seen. If children help, plan a small reward for them.

- Write out menus. Choose things that you or your family can put together easily. Casseroles, TV dinners, hot dogs, hamburgers, and meals that you have prepared and frozen ahead are all good ideas. Cook larger batches to be frozen so you will have them for future use. Add instructions so that other people can help you.

- Use shopping lists. Keep them handy so that they can be used as guides either by you or other people.

- When making casseroles for freezing, only partially cook rice and macaroni products. They will cook further in the reheating process. Add 1/2 cup liquid to refrigerated or frozen casseroles when reheating because they can get dry during refrigeration. Remember that frozen casseroles take a long time to heat completely—at least 45 minutes in deep dishes in the oven.

- Don't be shy about accepting gifts of food and offers of help from family and friends. Let them know what you like and offer your recipes. If people bring food you can't use right away, freeze it. That homecooked meal can break the monotony of quickie suppers. It also can save time when you're on a tight schedule. Date the food when you put it in the refrigerator or freezer.

- Have as few dishes, pots, and pans to wash as possible. Cook in dishes and pans that can also make attractive servers. Use paper napkins and disposable dishes, especially for dessert. Paper cups are fine for kids and for medicines. Disposable pans are a great timesaver—foil containers from frozen foods make good disposable pans. Soak dirty dishes to cut down washing time.

TABLE 1. SNACKS

Have these on hand for quick and easy nibbles:

Applesauce
Bread products, including muffins and crackers
Buttered popcorn
Cakes and cookies made with whole-grains, fruits, nuts, wheat germ, or granola
Cereal
Cheese, hard or semisoft
Cheesecake
Chocolate milk
Cottage cheese
Cream cheese and other soft cheese
Cream soups
Dips made with cheese, beans, or sour cream
Dried fruits, such as raisins, prunes, or apricots
Fruits (fresh or canned)
Gelatin salads and desserts
Granola
Hard-boiled and deviled eggs
Ice cream, frozen yogurt, popsicles
Juices
Milkshakes, instant breakfast drinks
Nuts
Peanut butter
Pizza
Puddings and custards
Quesadillas
Sandwiches
Vegetables (raw or cooked)
Yogurt (regular or frozen)

- When you are preparing soft dishes, choose foods that the whole family can eat, such as omelets, scrambled eggs, macaroni and cheese, meatloaf, tuna salad sandwiches, or tuna casseroles. Set aside enough food to be pureed in the blender or food processor for yourself.
- Use mixes, frozen ready-to-eat main dishes, and takeout foods whenever possible. The less time spent cooking and cleaning up, the more time for relaxation and the family.
- If someone is cooking for you, share this booklet with them for ideas for food selection and preparation. They will also get a better sense of your special needs.

Improving Your Nutrition

There are many ways to improve your nutrition to lessen the side effects of your treatment and to keep eating as well as you can when your treatment or illness is causing side effects. Table 1 provides a list of snacks you may want to try. Tables 2 and 3 on the following pages offer ideas for increasing protein and calories in your diet.

When side effects of treatment occur, they usually go away after treatment ends. Long-term treatment, however, may necessitate long-term changes in your diet to help you handle side effects and keep up your strength.

The ideas and suggestions listed here have worked for other cancer patients during their treatment. Each person is different, though, and you will have to find out what works best for you.

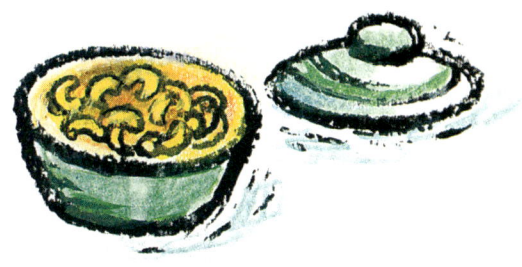

TABLE 2. HOW TO INCREASE PROTEIN

Hard or Semisoft Cheese	■ Melt on sandwiches, bread, muffins, tortillas, hamburgers, hot dogs, other meats or fish, vegetables, eggs, or desserts, such as stewed fruit or pies. ■ Grate and add to soups, sauces, casseroles, vegetable dishes, mashed potatoes, rice, noodles, or meatloaf.
Cottage Cheese/ Ricotta Cheese	■ Mix with or use to stuff fruits and vegetables. ■ Add to casseroles, spaghetti, noodles, and egg dishes, such as omelets, scrambled eggs, and souffles. ■ Use in gelatin, pudding-type desserts, cheesecake, and pancake batter. ■ Use to stuff crepes and pasta shells or manicotti.
Milk	■ Use milk in beverages and in cooking when possible. ■ Use in preparing hot cereal, soups, cocoa, and pudding. ■ Add cream sauces to vegetable and other dishes.
Powdered Milk	■ Add to regular milk and milk drinks, such as pasteurized eggnog and milkshakes. ■ Use in casseroles, meatloaf, breads, muffins, sauces, cream soups, mashed potatoes, puddings and custards, and milk-based desserts.
Commercial Products	■ See the section on "Commercial Products To Improve Nutrition" on page 45. ■ Use instant breakfast powder in milk drinks and desserts. ■ Mix with ice cream, milk, and fruit or flavorings for a high-protein milkshake.
Ice Cream, Yogurt, and Frozen Yogurt	■ Add to carbonated beverages, such as ginger ale; add to milk drinks, such as milkshakes. ■ Add to cereals, fruits, gelatin desserts, and pies; blend or whip with soft or cooked fruits. ■ Sandwich ice cream or frozen yogurt between enriched cake slices, cookies, or graham crackers.

TABLE 2. HOW TO INCREASE PROTEIN (continued)

Eggs	▪ Add chopped, hard-cooked eggs to salads and dressings, vegetables, casseroles, and creamed meats. ▪ Add extra eggs or egg whites to quiches and to pancake and French toast batter. Add extra egg whites to scrambled eggs and omelets. ▪ Make a rich custard with eggs, high-protein milk, and sugar. ▪ Add extra hard-cooked yolks to deviled-egg filling and sandwich spreads. ▪ *Avoid raw eggs, which may contain harmful bacteria, because your treatment may make you susceptible to infection.* Make sure all eggs you eat are well cooked or baked; avoid eggs that are "runny."
Nuts, Seeds, and Wheat Germ	▪ Add to casseroles, breads, muffins, pancakes, cookies, and waffles. ▪ Sprinkle on fruit, cereal, ice cream, yogurt, vegetables, salads, and toast as a crunchy topping; use in place of bread crumbs. ▪ Blend with parsley or spinach, herbs, and cream for a noodle, pasta, or vegetable sauce. ▪ Roll banana in chopped nuts.
Peanut Butter	▪ Spread on sandwiches, toast, muffins, crackers, waffles, pancakes, and fruit slices. ▪ Use as a dip for raw vegetables such as carrots, cauliflower, and celery. ▪ Blend with milk drinks and beverages. ▪ Swirl through soft ice cream and yogurt.
Meat and Fish	▪ Add chopped, cooked meat or fish to vegetables, salads, casseroles, soups, sauces, and biscuit dough. ▪ Use in omelets, souffles, quiches, sandwich fillings, and chicken and turkey stuffings. ▪ Wrap in piecrust or biscuit dough as turnovers. ▪ Add to stuffed baked potatoes.
Beans/Legumes	▪ Cook and use dried peas, legumes, beans, and bean curd (tofu) in soups or add to casseroles, pastas, and grain dishes that also contain cheese or meat. Mash with cheese and milk.

\multicolumn{2}{c}{*TABLE 3.* HOW TO INCREASE CALORIES}
Butter and Margarine	■ Add to soups, mashed and baked potatoes, hot cereals, grits, rice, noodles, and cooked vegetables. ■ Stir into cream soups, sauces, and gravies. ■ Combine with herbs and seasonings, and spread on cooked meats, hamburgers, and fish and egg dishes. ■ Use melted butter or margarine as a dip for raw vegetables and seafoods, such as shrimp, scallops, crab, and lobster.
Whipped Cream	■ Use sweetened on hot chocolate, desserts, gelatin, puddings, fruits, pancakes, and waffles. ■ Fold unsweetened into mashed potatoes or vegetable purees.
Table Cream	■ Use in cream soups, sauces, egg dishes, batters, puddings, and custards. ■ Put on hot or cold cereal. ■ Mix with noodles, pasta, rice, and mashed potatoes. ■ Pour on chicken and fish while baking. ■ Use as a binder in hamburgers, meatloaf, and croquettes. ■ Add to milk in recipes. ■ Make hot chocolate with cream and add marshmallows.
Cream Cheese	■ Spread on breads, muffins, fruit slices, and crackers. ■ Add to vegetables. ■ Roll into balls and coat with chopped nuts, wheat germ, or granola.
Sour Cream	■ Add to cream soups, baked potatoes, macaroni and cheese, vegetables, sauces, salad dressings, stews, baked meat, and fish. ■ Use as a topping for cakes, fruit, gelatin desserts, breads, and muffins. ■ Use as a dip for fresh fruits and vegetables. ■ For a good dessert, scoop it on fresh fruit, add brown sugar, and let it sit in the refrigerator for a while.

TABLE 3. HOW TO INCREASE CALORIES (continued)

Salad Dressings and Mayonnaise	▪ Spread on sandwiches and crackers. ▪ Combine with meat, fish, and egg or vegetable salads. ▪ Use as a binder in croquettes. ▪ Use in sauces and gelatin dishes.
Honey, Jam, and Sugar	▪ Add to bread, cereal, milk drinks, and fruit and yogurt desserts. ▪ Use as a glaze for meats, such as chicken.
Granola	▪ Use in cookie, muffin, and bread batters. ▪ Sprinkle on vegetables, yogurt, ice cream, pudding, custard, and fruit. ▪ Layer with fruits and bake. ▪ Mix with dry fruits and nuts for a snack. ▪ Substitute for bread or rice in pudding recipes.
Dried Fruits	▪ Cook and serve for breakfast or as a dessert or snack. ▪ Add to muffins, cookies, breads, cakes, rice and grain dishes, cereals, puddings, and stuffings. ▪ Bake in pies and turnovers. ▪ Combine with cooked vegetables, such as carrots, sweet potatoes, yams, and acorn and butternut squash. ▪ Combine with nuts or granola for snacks.
Eggs	▪ Add chopped, hard-cooked eggs to salads and dressings, vegetables, casseroles, and creamed meats. ▪ Make a rich custard with eggs, milk, and sugar. ▪ Add extra, hard-cooked yolks to deviled-egg filling and sandwich spread. ▪ Beat eggs into mashed potatoes, vegetable purees, and sauces. *(Be sure to keep cooking these dishes after adding the eggs because raw eggs may contain harmful bacteria.)* ▪ Add extra eggs or egg whites to custards, puddings, quiches, scrambled eggs, omelets, and to pancake and French toast batter before cooking.
Food Preparation	▪ Bread, meats and vegetables. ▪ Sauté and fry foods when possible, because these cooking methods add more calories than baking or broiling. ▪ Add sauces or gravies.

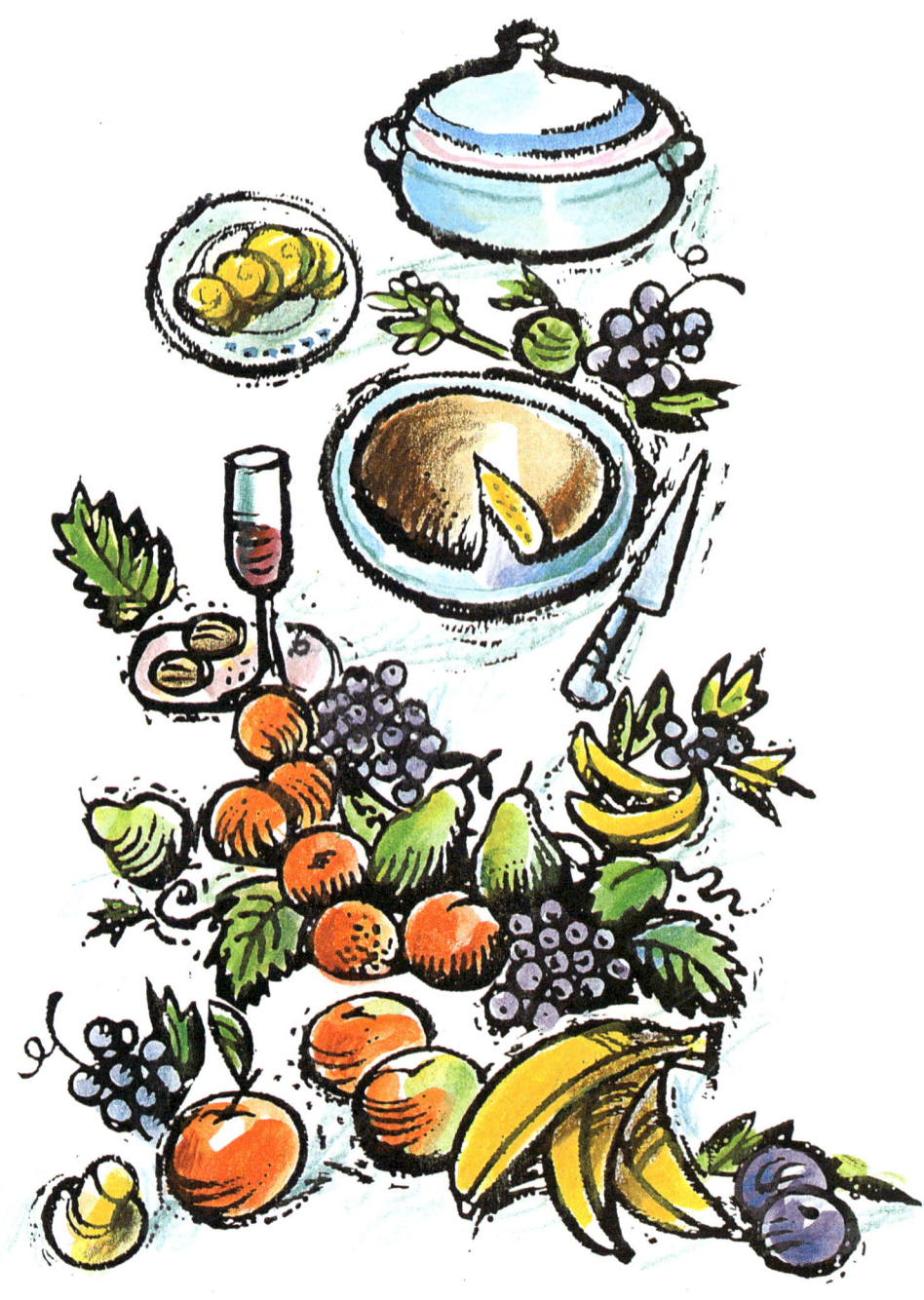

Special Diets For Special Needs

When you have special needs because of your illness or treatment, your doctor or registered dietitian may prescribe a special diet. They also may suggest a commercial product to help you meet your nutritional needs. In the following sections, you will find guidelines for several special diets used during cancer treatment. You also will learn about products that can boost nutrition and where you can buy them. *Remember that special diets and products to improve nutrition should be used only as recommended by your doctor or registered dietitian.*

Special diets are an important tool for correcting nutritional problems that occur during cancer treatment. For example, a soft diet may be best if your mouth, throat, esophagus, or stomach is sore. Or, if your treatment makes it difficult for you to digest dairy products, you may need to follow a low-lactose diet. Some diets are well balanced and can be followed for long periods of time. However, some special diets should be followed for only a few days because they may not provide enough nutrients for the long term.

Only your doctor or registered dietitian should decide whether you need a special diet and for how long. If you are already following a special diet for another health problem, such as diabetes or high cholesterol, you and your doctor and registered dietitian should work together to develop your new plan.

Guidelines for common special diets appear in this section, including:

- Clear-liquid diet.
- Full-liquid diet.
- Soft diet.
- Fiber-restricted diet.
- Low-lactose diet.

For each diet, you will find a brief explanation of when the diet usually is recommended, the major foods it includes, and a suggested meal pattern. This information will help you follow the diet recommended by your doctor or registered dietitian. If you think you need a special diet, talk with your doctor or registered dietitian.

\multicolumn{3}{c}{**CLEAR-LIQUID DIET**}
Type of Food	**Allowed Items**	**Excluded Items**
Beverages	Water; carbonated beverages; cereal beverages; coffee, tea;* fruit-flavored drinks; strained lemonade, limeade, and fruit punches	Milk, milk drinks, all others**
Breads Cereals Flours	None	All
Cheeses	None	All
Desserts	Plain gelatin desserts, fruit ices without milk or pieces of fruit, popsicles	All others
Eggs	None	All
Fats	None	All

*Your doctor may recommend decaffeinated coffee or tea.
**Check with your doctor about alcohol. Alcohol cannot be used safely with some medicines.

Clear-Liquid Diet

Clear-liquid diets are useful if the body can't handle the softest foods or heavy or thick liquids. Patients usually follow this type of diet after surgery or before stomach or bowel surgery. Patients with severe nausea and vomiting may also have this diet. A clear-liquid diet often lasts 1 to 2 days or until you can drink or eat other beverages and foods. It cannot meet the daily servings suggested on page 4 (except for fruit juices), but it helps ensure that your body doesn't lose too much fluid as you recover and become ready for a regular diet.

CLEAR-LIQUID DIET (continued)

Type of Food	Allowed Items	Excluded items
Fruits **Fruit Juices**	Apple, cranberry, and grape juice; strained citrus juices if tolerated	All others
Meat **Poultry** **Fish** **Legumes**	None	All
Milk **Milk Products**	None	All
Potatoes **Rice** **Pasta**	None	All
Soup	Bouillon, clear fat-free broths, consommé	All others
Sweets	Honey, jelly, syrups, plain sugar candy in small amounts	All others
Vegetables	Strained vegetable broth	All others
Miscellaneous	Salt	All others

CLEAR-LIQUID DIET *Suggested Meal Pattern*

Breakfast

1 cup juice
1 cup clear broth
1/2 cup gelatin dessert
Coffee or tea* with sugar

Snack

1 cup fruit juice or soft drink
1/2 cup gelatin dessert

Lunch

1 cup juice
1 cup clear broth
1/2 cup gelatin dessert
Coffee or tea* with sugar

Snack

1 cup fruit juice or soft drink
1/2 cup gelatin dessert

Dinner

1 cup juice
1 cup clear broth
1/2 cup gelatin dessert
Coffee or tea* with sugar

Snack

1 cup fruit juice or soft drink
1/2 cup gelatin dessert

FULL-LIQUID DIET		
Type of Food	**Allowed Items**	**Excluded Items**
Beverages	Cereal beverages; coffee, tea:* fruit drinks; strained lemonade, limeade, or fruit punches; water	None**
Breads Cereals Flours	Refined or strained cooked cereal	Breads and cereals in solid form
Cheeses	Cheese soup	All others
Desserts	Plain gelatin desserts, junket, soft or baked custards, sherbets, plain cornstarch pudding, fresh or frozen yogurt, ice milk, smooth ice cream	All others, particularly those with fruits or seeds
Eggs	Pasteurized eggnog	All others
Fats	Butter, cream, oils, margarine	All others
Fruits Fruit Juices	All juices and nectars, thin fruit purees	All others

* *Your doctor may recommend decaffeinated coffee or tea.*
** *Check with your doctor before drinking alcohol. Alcohol cannot be used safely with some medicines.*

Full-Liquid Diet

You may follow a full-liquid diet when your body can digest all liquids but can't handle solid food yet. Your doctor or registered dietitian may recommend this diet after surgery or when you can't chew and swallow food. All liquids served at room or body temperature are part of this diet. This diet can include most of the recommended food groups on pages 4 and 5, except meat. Extra milk has been included to ensure adequate protein. When planned properly, this diet can be used for long periods. In these instances, your doctor may prescribe a commercial supplement and/or certain vitamins. However, you should only take these if your doctor or registered dietitian recommends them.

FULL-LIQUID DIET (continued)

Type of Food	Allowed Items	Excluded Items
Meat **Poultry** **Fish** **Legumes**	Small amounts of strained meat in broth or gelatin	All others
Milk **Milk Products**	Buttermilk and chocolate, skim, and whole milk; ice milk; milkshakes; plain yogurt	All others, yogurt with pieces of fruit
Potatoes **Rice** **Pasta**	Potatoes pureed in soup	All others
Soups	Bouillon, broth, clear cream soups, any strained or blenderized soup	All others
Sweets	Honey, jelly, syrups in small amounts	All others
Vegetables	Tomato puree for cream soups; tomato, vegetable juices	All others
Miscellaneous	Flavoring extracts, salt	All others

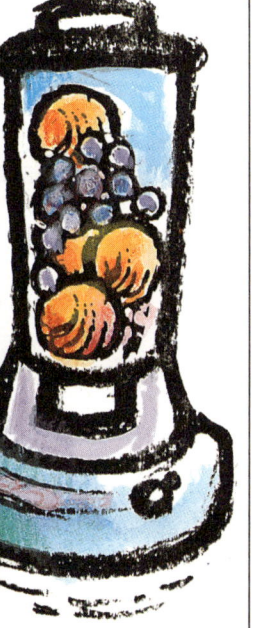

FULL-LIQUID DIET *Suggested Meal Pattern*

Breakfast

1 cup fruit juice
1 cup strained cereal
1 cup milk
Coffee or tea* with sugar

Snack
1 cup fruit juice

Lunch

1 cup strained soup, (made with vegetable purée)
1 cup strained cereal
1/2 cup allowed dessert
1 cup fruit juice
1 cup milk or yogurt
Coffee or tea* with sugar

Snack

1 cup milk or eggnog

Dinner

1 cup strained cream soup (with a small amount of strained meat)
1 cup milk
1 cup strained cereal
1/2 cup allowed dessert
1 cup vegetable juice
Coffee or tea* with sugar

Snack

1 cup milk or yogurt

If you must follow a full-liquid diet over a long period, you can increase the protein and calorie content of the diet by:

- Adding nonfat dry milk to beverages and soups.
- Adding instant breakfast powder to milk, puddings, custards, and milkshakes.
- Adding strained meats (such as those in baby food) to broths.

You can increase the calories of a full-liquid diet by:

- Adding butter to hot cereal and soups.
- Including sugar or syrup (glucose) in beverages.
- Using smooth ice cream in desserts and beverages.
- Using prepared breakfast mixes in milk or milkshakes.

You will find other helpful ideas in Table 2 "How To Increase Protein" and Table 3 "How To Increase Calories" in the section "Improving Your Nutrition." These tables begin on page 24.

Soft Diet

A soft diet is useful when your body is ready for more than liquids but still unable to handle a regular solid diet. Soft food is easier to eat than regular food when the mouth, throat, esophagus, and/or stomach are sore. This soreness can occur to these parts of the body during and after radiation therapy or during chemotherapy. A soft diet can be used for long periods because it contains all needed nutrients. The diet consists of bland, lower fat foods that you soften by cooking, mashing, puréeing, or blending.

The table on the next two pages lists foods included in a soft diet as well as foods you should try to avoid. Keep in mind, however, that you may be able to eat some of the "excluded" foods without any discomfort or problems. In general, though, it is probably best to avoid fried or greasy foods and foods that may cause gas.

SOFT DIET

Type of Food	Allowed Items	Excluded Items
Beverages	All	None**
Breads	French, Vienna, Italian, seedless rye, white, refined whole wheat, cornbread, or any except whole-grain; if tolerated, muffins, French toast, crackers, biscuits, rolls, pancakes, waffles	Brown, cracked wheat, pumpernickel, raisin, rye with seeds, buckwheat; whole-grain crackers; rolls with coconut, raisins, nuts, or whole grains; tortillas
Cereals	Refined, cooked, or ready-to-eat, such as cream of wheat, farina, hominy grits, cornmeal, oatmeal, puffed rice	Whole-grain or bran
Flours	All except those excluded	Whole-grain, bran, or wheat
Cheeses	All except those excluded	Sharp or strongly flavored cheeses; those containing whole seeds and spices
Desserts	Ice milk, ice cream, sherbet, ices, custards, gelatins, or others with allowed fruits	Desserts made with excluded fruits, nuts, coconut
Eggs	All except those excluded	Raw, fried
Fats	Butter, cream, cream substitutes, vegetable shortening and oils, margarine, mayonnaise, sour cream, commercial French dressing	Other salad dressings; salt pork; fried foods
Fruits **Fruit Juices**	All juices and nectars; avocado, banana, canned or cooked apples, apricots, cherries, grapefruit and orange sections without membrane, peaches, pears, seedless grapes, tomatoes; soft melons, such as watermelon, if tolerated	All raw fruit except avocado and banana; all dried fruit; berries, crabapples, coconut, figs, grapes, pineapples, plums, rhubarb
Meat	Tender beef, lamb, veal, or liver that is baked, broiled, creamed, roasted, or stewed; roasted or stewed pork	Fried, salted, and smoked meats; chitterlings; corned beef; sausage; cold cuts

** *Check with your doctor before drinking alcohol. Alcohol cannot be used safely with some medicines.*

SOFT DIET (continued)

Type of Food	Allowed items	Excluded Items
Poultry	Chicken, Cornish game hen, turkey, chicken livers	Duck, goose; fried poultry
Fish	Cooked, fresh, or frozen fish without bones; tuna, salmon	Fried fish, shellfish, anchovies, caviar, herring, sardines, snails, skate
Legumes **Nuts**	Creamy peanut butter	All other legumes, nuts, and seed kernels
Milk **Milk Products**	All	None
Potatoes **Rice** **Pasta**	Baked, boiled, creamed, scalloped, mashed, au gratin; mashed sweet potatoes; dumplings; noodles; brown or white rice; spaghetti	French fries, hashbrowns, potato salad, whole sweet potatoes or yams; bread stuffing; fritters; chow mein noodles; wild rice; barley
Soups	Bouillon, broth, consommé, strained cream and vegetable	Bean, split pea, onion; bisques; gumbos; unstrained chowders
Sweets	Apple butter, butterscotch candy, caramels, chocolate, fondant, plain fudge, lollipops, marshmallows, mints, honey, jelly, syrups, sugars in small amounts	Candied fruits, nut brittle, jams, preserves, marmalade, marzipan, fruit sauces with prohibited fruits
Vegetables	Canned or cooked asparagus, carrots, beets, eggplant, mushrooms, parsley, pumpkin, spinach, squash, vegetable juice cocktail, raw lettuce if tolerated	All raw vegetables except lettuce; all canned or cooked vegetables not specifically listed as allowed
Miscellaneous	Aspic, catsup, gelatin, gravy, pretzels, soy sauce, vinegar; brown, cheese, cream, tomato, and white sauces; all finely chopped or ground leaf herbs and spices	Garlic, horseradish; olives, pickles; popcorn, potato chips; relishes; chili, a-la-king, creole, barbecue, cocktail, sweet-and-sour, Newburg, and Worcestershire sauces; whole and seed herbs and spices

SOFT DIET *Suggested Meal Pattern*

Breakfast

1/2 cup fruit or juice
2 eggs, scrambled
1 slice toast
1 tsp. butter or margarine
Jelly
Sugar and cream
Beverage

Snack

1/2 to 1 cup cereal
1 cup milk
Sugar

Lunch

1/2 cup fruit juice
2 oz. meat, fish, or poultry
1/2 cup vegetable
2 slices bread
1 tsp. butter or margarine
1 cup milk

Snack

Banana
2 tbsp. creamy peanut butter

Dinner

4 oz. meat, fish, or poultry
1 cup potato
1/2 cup vegetable
1 slice bread or roll
1 tsp. butter or margarine
1 serving fruit or
   allowed dessert
Beverage

Snack

1/2 cup fruit or allowed dessert
1 cup milk, milkshake, or
   pasteurized eggnog

Fiber-Restricted

Your doctor or registered dietitian may recommend a fiber-restricted diet if your **gastrointestinal (GI)** tract cannot digest fiber in foods. This type of diet is often used after GI surgery before patients return to their regular diet. A fiber-restricted diet also may be needed when treatment, such as radiation, damages the bowel or when the GI tract becomes irritated.

A fiber-restricted diet limits the amount of vegetables, fruits, cereals, and grains that you can eat. It also limits to two cups per day the amount of milk and milk products, such as cream, yogurt, and cheese, that you can eat. Milk does not contain fiber, but it leaves a residue in the GI tract that can irritate the bowel and cause diarrhea and cramping. The diet also is helpful for the many cancer patients who have a hard time digesting the milk sugar, lactose. (See the section, "Low-Lactose Diet," on pages 41-43.) A fiber-restricted diet can be changed easily, depending on how you feel after eating certain foods. Use the diet in this booklet as a guide and discuss any changes with your doctor or registered dietitian.

There may be times when a low-residue diet, which is more limited than a fiber-restricted diet, is needed. On the low-residue diet, you may be able to eat most strained vegetables and fruit juices, such as white potatoes without skin, and tomato juice. All other forms of vegetables and fruits may be excluded from the diet. The low-residue diet also limits the amount of fat and dairy products you can eat. Your doctor or registered dietitian will let you know if you need to follow a low-residue diet.

Your registered dietitian may gradually increase fiber and milk products in your diet according to how well you handle them.

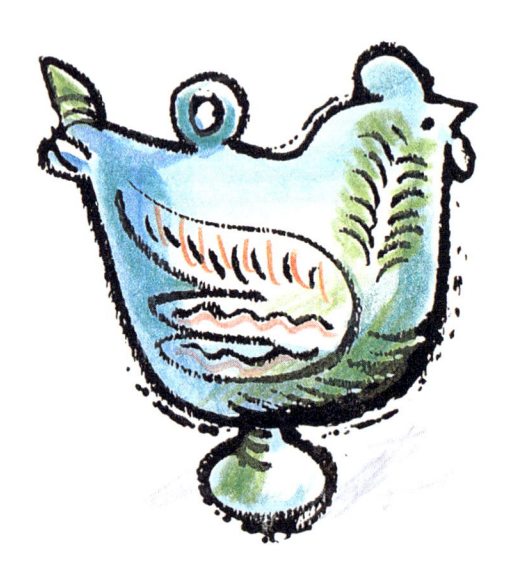

FIBER-RESTRICTED DIET

Type of Food	Allowed Items	Excluded Items
Beverages	Fruit-flavored drinks; carbonated beverages, coffee, tea;* milk drinks and milk used in cooking (2 cups milk or milk products allowed per day, if tolerated); all others except excluded items, no limitations	Prune juice, pear nectar**
Breads	French, Vienna, Italian, refined wheat, white, and rye breads without seeds; crackers; biscuits; French toast; plain hard crust; zwieback rolls	Breads, crackers, rolls, or cereals containing whole grain or graham flour; bran, seeds, nuts, or raisins; cornbread
Cereals	All refined, cooked, or dry cereals, such as cream of wheat or rice and flaked or puffed cereals	All whole-grain cereals made from prohibited flours or other foods; oatmeal; granola
Cheeses	Cottage, cream, American, Swiss, Muenster, or other mild cheese; 1 oz. may be substituted for 1 cup milk	All others
Desserts	Custards, gelatin puddings, plain cookies and cakes, sherbets; 1/2 cup ice cream (may be substituted as 1/2 cup milk allowance), pastries made with allowed ingredients	All desserts containing seeds, nuts, coconut, or raisins; tough-skinned fruits
Eggs	All except raw	Raw
Fats	Butter, oils, cream, dry cream substitutes, margarine, mayonnaise, shortenings, smooth salad dressings, sour cream	Salad dressing made with excluded foods; tartar sauce
Fruits	Canned or cooked fruits without seeds, skins, or membranes — apples, applesauce, cherries, grapefruit, oranges, tangerine, peaches, pineapple, pears, fruit cocktail; raw — ripe bananas, melon, grapefruit, oranges, tangerine; juice — all except prune juice and pear nectar (2 servings allowed per day)	All other fruits; dried fruits; berries; figs; grapes with seeds; stewed prunes, prune purée; plums; pear nectar

*Your doctor may recommend decaffeinated coffee or tea.
**Check with your doctor before drinking alcohol. Alcohol cannot be used safely with some medicines.

FIBER-RESTRICTED DIET (Continued)

Type of Food	Allowed Items	Excluded Items
Meat **Poultry**	Tender beef, ham, lamb, liver, poultry, or veal that is baked, broiled, or stewed; lean or low-fat cold cuts and frankfurters	Fried meats and poultry, smoked or cured meats, cold cuts, corned beef, frankfurters, pastrami, sausage
Fish	Fresh or frozen fish without bones, canned tuna or salmon, cooked shellfish	All fried or smoked fish, sardines, herring
Legumes **Nuts**	None	All dried legumes, lima beans, peas, nuts
Milk **Milk Products**	Buttermilk and chocolate, skim, low-fat, and whole milk, if tolerated; yogurt, plain, custard-style, with allowed fruits and without nuts (2 cups, including that used in cooking, allowed per day)	Yogurt containing fruits
Potatoes **Rice** **Pasta**	Boiled, creamed, mashed, and scalloped potatoes without skin; macaroni, noodles, white rice, spaghetti (1 serving potato allowed per day; all others, no limitation)	Potato skin, potato cakes, french fries, hash browns, potato salad, sweet potato, brown and wild rice, barley, hominy
Soups	Cream and broth-based soups made with allowed foods	All others
Sweets	Honey, jelly, syrup, plain hard candy, molasses, marshmallows, gumdrops	Jams, preserves, candies with fruits, coconut, raisins, nuts, candied fruits
Vegetables	Canned or cooked asparagus tips, green or wax beans, mushrooms, peas, pumpkin, raw lettuce, if tolerated (no limitation on vegetable juices; 1 serving whole vegetables allowed per day)	All raw vegetables except lettuce; canned or cooked vegetables not specifically allowed, such as the high-fiber vegetables: beans, carrots, peas, spinach and other greens, beets
Miscellaneous	Ground or finely chopped herbs and spices, salt, flavoring extracts, catsup, chocolate, mild gravy, white sauce, soy sauce, vinegar	All other spices and condiments, olives, pickles, potato chips, popcorn

FIBER RESTRICTED DIET *Suggested Meal Pattern*

Breakfast

1/2 cup strained fruit juice*
1 egg
1 slice white toast
3 tsp. butter or margarine
Jelly

Snack

1 cup milk**
1 serving allowed cereal
Sugar

Lunch

1/2 cup soup***
2 oz. meat, poultry, or fish
1/2 cup allowed vegetable
2 slices white bread or roll
1 serving allowed dessert

Snack

2 slices white toast
2 tsp. butter or margarine
Jelly or honey

Dinner

5 oz. meat, poultry, or fish
1 cup milk**
3 tsp. butter or margarine
1 baked potato, without skin
1 serving allowed dessert
1/2 cup vegetable juice

Snack

1/2 cup strained fruit juice*
3 plain cookies

* 2 servings of fruit/juices allowed per day.
** 2 servings of milk allowed per day.
*** Count as 1/2 cup milk if made with milk.

Low-Lactose Diet

All milk products contain lactose (or milk sugar). The doctor or registered dietitian may recommend a low-lactose diet after radiation therapy to the intestines, which often makes lactose hard to digest for a time. Fermented milk products, such as buttermilk, acidophilus milk, sour cream, and yogurt, usually are easier to handle than whole milk. You also can buy low-lactose milk or use liquid drops or caplets that help break down the lactose in milk and other dairy products. Lactose is often used as a filler in many products such as instant coffee and some medicines. Carefully read labels on commercial foods to see if they contain lactose or any milk products or milk solids.

Lactose tolerance varies from person to person. Ask your doctor or registered dietitian about choosing allowed foods and about low-lactose dairy products that you can buy at the grocery store.

LOW-LACTOSE DIET

Type of Food	Allowed Items	Excluded Items
Beverages	Water, lactose-free carbonated beverages, fruit-flavored drinks, fruit punches, lemonade, limeade, nondairy product drinks, low-lactose milk, acidophilus milk, coffee, and tea*	Artificial fruit drinks containing lactose, all beverages and nutritional supplements made with milk and milk products with the exception of buttermilk, low-lactose milk, and yogurt**
Bread	All	None
Cereals	Any cooked or dry cereal not containing lactose	Instant hot cereals, high-protein cereals, all cereals with added milk or lactose
Flours	All	None
Cheeses	Fermented cheeses (cheddar and any cheese aged with bacteria)	All others
Desserts	Fruit ices; gelatins; angel food cake; desserts made with nondairy products, buttermilk, or sour cream	Ice cream, puddings, and other desserts containing milk or milk products
Eggs	All except raw eggs and eggs prepared with milk or milk products	Creamed, scrambled, omelets, or other eggs prepared with milk; raw eggs
Fats	Margarine not containing milk solids, vegetable oils, mayonnaise, shortening	All others: cream, half-and-half, table and whipping cream, butter
Fruits **Fruit Juices**	All fresh, canned, or frozen fruit juices; fruits not processed with lactose	Any canned or frozen fruits and fruit juices processed with lactose
Meat **Poultry** **Fish** **Legumes** **Nuts**	Any except those specifically excluded	Creamed or breaded fish, poultry, meat; cold cuts, hot dogs, liver, sausage, or other processed meats containing milk or lactose; gravies made with milk

* *Your doctor may recommend decaffeinated coffee or tea.*
** *Check with your doctor before drinking alcohol. Alcohol cannot be used safely with some medicines.*

LOW-LACTOSE DIET (Continued)

Type of Food	Allowed Items	Excluded Items
Milk **Milk Products**	Fermented milk products such as acidophilus milk, buttermilk, yogurt, and sour cream; low-lactose products; "lactose-digesting" pills or caplets	All milk, milk products except those allowed
Potatoes **Rice** **Pasta**	White or sweet potatoes, macaroni, noodles, spaghetti or other pasta, rice	Any prepared with milk, such as commercially prepared creamed or scalloped potato products containing dried milk
Soups	Broth-based soups	Cream soups, chowders, commercially prepared soups that contain milk or milk products
Sweets	Honey, jams, preserves, syrups, molasses	Candy containing lactose, milk, or cocoa; butterscotch candies; caramels; chocolates (Read all labels carefully.)
Vegetables	All vegetables except those prepared with milk	Any prepared with milk, such as creamed, scalloped, or any processed vegetables containing lactose
Miscellaneous	Catsup, chili sauce, horseradish, olives, pickles, vinegar, gravies prepared without milk, mustard, all herbs and spices, peanut butter, unbuttered popcorn	Chocolate, cocoa, milk gravies, cream sauces, chewing gum, instant coffee, powdered soft drinks, artificial juices containing milk or lactose

LOW-LACTOSE DIET *Suggested Meal Pattern*

Breakfast

1/2 cup fruit juice
1 serving cereal
1 slice toast
1 tsp. margarine*
Jelly
1 cup acidophilus or
 low-lactose milk
Sugar
Salt and pepper
Beverage

Snack

Crackers*
2 tbsp. peanut butter
Jelly or honey

Lunch

3 oz. meat or substitute
1/2 cup vegetable and/or salad
2 slices bread or roll
2 tsp. margarine*
1 serving fruit
Salt and pepper
Beverage

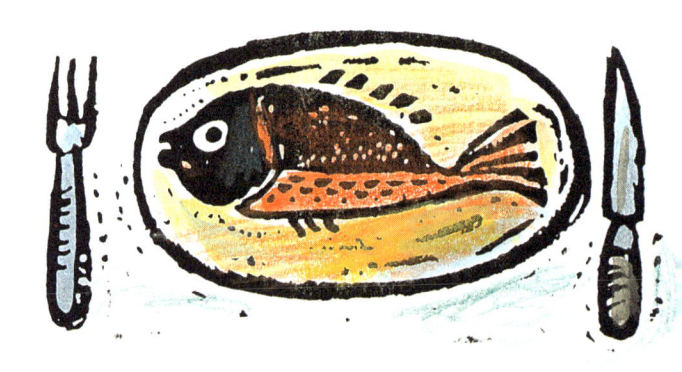

* Should not contain milk solids.

Snack

Broth-based soup
1 slice bread or roll
1 tsp. margarine*

Dinner

1 serving salad
3 oz. meat or substitute
1/2 cup rice
1/2 cup vegetable
1 serving fruit or dessert
1 cup acidophilus or
 low-lactose milk
Salt and pepper

Snack

1/2 cup juice
Popcorn or pretzels*

Commercial Products To Improve Nutrition

If you cannot get enough calories and protein from your diet, commercial nutrition supplements, such as formulas and instant breakfast powders, may be helpful. There also are products that can be added to any food or beverage to boost calorie content. These supplements are high in protein and calories and have extra vitamins and minerals. They come in liquid, pudding, and powder forms. Prepackaged blenderized diets made from whole foods also are available. These are a convenient and inexpensive alternative to homemade preparations. Most commercial nutrition supplements contain little or no lactose. However, it is important to check the label if you are sensitive to lactose. (See the section, "Low-Lactose Diet," on pages 41-43.)

These products need no refrigeration until you open them. Thus, you can carry nutrition supplements with you and take them whenever you feel hungry or thirsty. They are good chilled as between-meal and bedtime snacks. You may want to take a can or two with you when you go for treatments or other times when long waits may tire you. Ask your registered dietitian which supplements would be best for you.

Many supermarkets and drugstores carry a variety of commercial nutrition supplements. If you don't see these products on the shelf, ask the store manager if they can be ordered. You also may want to ask your doctor or registered dietitian for information about products for special patients. Be sure to ask for manufacturers' names, and, as mentioned above, be sure to read the label to see if any of the products contains lactose.

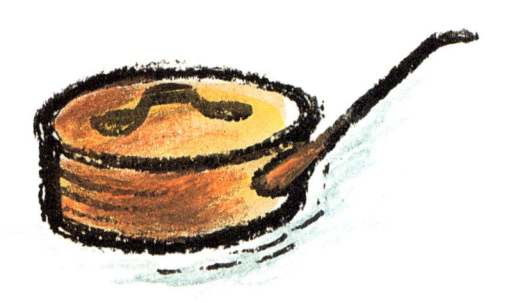

RESOURCES

Information about cancer is available from many sources, including the ones listed below. For additional information you may wish to check the local library, bookstores, or support groups in your community.

Cancer Information Service

The Cancer Information Service, a program of the National Cancer Institute, is a nationwide telephone service for cancer patients and their families and friends, the public, and health care professionals. The staff can answer questions (in English or Spanish) and can send free National Cancer Institute materials about cancer. They also know about support groups and other resources and services. One toll-free number, 1-800-4-CANCER (1-800-422-6237), connects callers with the office that serves their area.

American Cancer Society

The American Cancer Society is a voluntary organization with local units all over the country. This organization supports research, conducts educational programs, and offers support groups and many other services to patients and their families. The American Cancer Society also provides free booklets. To obtain booklets or for information about services and activities in local areas, call the toll-free number 1-800-ACS-2345 (1-800-227-2345), or the number listed under American Cancer Society in the white pages of the telephone book.

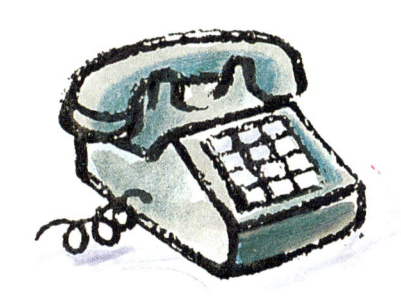

GLOSSARY

Anorexia: Loss of appetite for food.

Antiemetic: A drug used to control nausea and vomiting.

Biological therapy (immunotherapy): Treatment to stimulate or restore the ability of the immune system to fight infection and disease. This treatment uses products from the body's natural defense system to destroy cancer cells.

Calorie: Calories measure the energy your body gets from food. Your body needs calories as "fuel" to perform all of its functions, such as breathing, circulating the blood, and physical activity. When you are sick, your body may need extra calories to fight fever or other problems.

Carbohydrate: One of the three nutrients that supply calories (energy) to the body. Carbohydrates are needed for normal body function. There are two basic kinds of carbohydrates: simple (sugars) and complex (starches and fiber).

Chemotherapy: The use of drugs to stop cancer cells from growing in size or number.

Dehydration: When the body loses too much water to work well. Severe diarrhea or vomiting can cause dehydration.

Diet: The food you eat, including both liquids and solids.

Dietary fat: One of the three nutrients that supply calories (energy) to the body. Fat also helps the body absorb certain vitamins. Small amounts of fat are necessary for normal body function. Foods high in fat are also high in calories.

Diuretics: Drugs that help the body get rid of water and salt.

Dyspepsia/indigestion: Upset stomach.

Dysphagia: Difficulty in swallowing.

Edema: The buildup of excess fluid within the tissues.

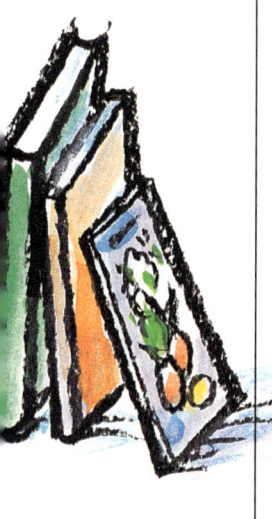

47

Electrolytes: A general term for the minerals necessary to give the body the proper fluid balance.

Fortified: A food is fortified when extra nutrients are added.

Gastrointestinal (GI): Having to do with the digestive tract, which includes the mouth, esophagus, stomach, and intestines.

Glucose: A simple sugar occurring in some fruits and honey; the sugar found in blood.

Immunotherapy: See biological therapy.

Infection: When germs enter the body and produce disease, the disease is called an infection. Infections can occur in any part of the body. They cause a fever and other problems, depending on the site of the infection. When the body's natural defense system is strong, it can often fight the entering germs and prevent infection. Cancer treatment can weaken the natural defense system, but good nutrition can help make it stronger.

Intravenous (IV) feeding: When a person receives some of the nutrients he or she needs through a needle in a vein. IV feeding occurs when a person is unable to eat solid food, such as right after surgery.

Lactose intolerance: Lactose is a sugar in milk. After some types of surgery you may no longer be able to digest lactose easily. This lactose intolerance may go away over time. There are special milk products without lactose.

Malnutrition: When the body receives too few of the essential nutrients.

Minerals: Nutrients required by the body in small amounts such as iron, calcium, and potassium.

Nutrient: The part of the food you eat that the body uses to grow, function, and stay alive. The major classes of nutrients that the body needs are proteins, carbohydrates, minerals, fats, and vitamins.

Nutrition: A three-part process that gives the body the nutrients it needs. First, you eat or drink food. Second, the body breaks the food down into nutrients. Third, the nutrients travel through the bloodstream to different parts of the body where they are used as "fuel." To give your body proper nutrition, you have to eat or drink enough of the foods that contain key nutrients.

Potassium: A mineral the body needs for fluid balance and other essential functions.

Protein: One of the three nutrients that supply calories (energy) to the body. The protein we eat becomes a part of our muscle, bone, skin, and blood.

Radiation therapy: Treatment with high-energy x-rays to kill or damage cancer cells. External radiation therapy is the use of a machine to aim high-energy x-rays at the cancer. Internal radiation therapy is the placement of radioactive material inside the body as close as possible to the cancer.

Registered dietitian: A professional who plans diet programs for proper nutrition.

Sodium: A mineral required by the body to keep body fluids in balance; too much sodium can cause you to retain water.

Total parenteral nutrition (TPN): When a person receives all of the nutrients needed through a needle in a vein. TPN may be used when the mouth, the stomach, or the bowel are sore from cancer treatment.

Vitamins: Key nutrients that the body needs to grow and stay strong. The best sources of vitamins, such as vitamins A, B, and C, are the foods we eat.

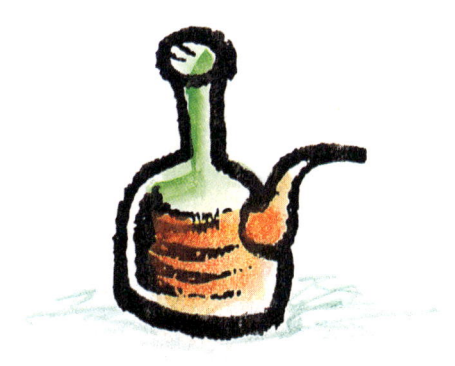

Recipes for Better Nutrition During Cancer Treatment

The recipes were especially chosen to help solve the problems discussed in this book. To be included, the recipes also had to be high in nutritional value, easy to make, good tasting, and useable for the family as well as for the patient. You will find some old favorites—but calories, protein, or other nutrients have been added. All of the recipes have been taste-tested, and only the favorites from the taste-testing have been included.

At the bottom of each recipe is a chart that gives information about the recipe's protein and calorie content as well as its suitability for the special requirements of cancer patients. Shading is used in two ways:

- If shading occurs in a box below "SPECIAL DIETS," it means the recipe is particularly good for that specific diet. If an asterisk appears in one of these boxes, the recipe can be adjusted as indicated in the footnote to make it suitable for that diet.

- If shading occurs in the protein and/or calorie box, the recipe is a rich source of these.

For example, the chart below shows a recipe good for a patient on a low-lactose diet and one rich in protein but not particularly high in calories.

		SPECIAL DIETS			
Calories per SV	Protein g/ SV	Full-Liquid	Soft	Fiber-Restricted	Low-Lactose
160	12				

Abbreviations: In all recipes, **tsp.** is teaspoon, **tbsp.** is tablespoon, **oz.** is ounce, and **lb.** is pound; **SV** is serving. All temperatures are °F.

Note: Some recipes use specific ingredients, such as soy-based nutritional supplements. You may want to try different product brands to see which ones taste best to you. You also can ask a registered dietitian for more helpful suggestions.

Soft, moist, and nourishing, this recipe is just as popular with or without milk.

Macaroni and Cheese

1 cup milk
1 tbsp. flour
1-2 tbsp. margarine
1 tsp. minced onion
salt and pepper to taste

1 tsp. dry mustard (optional)
2 cups elbow macaroni, cooked
  and drained
1 cup shredded cheddar cheese

Measure milk into the pan and blend in flour until no lumps remain. Add margarine, onion, and other seasonings and cook until sauce thickens. Stir in macaroni and cheese. Bake uncovered in greased, 1-quart casserole at 400° for 15 minutes or until slightly browned and bubbly. May be frozen before baking. Serves 4.

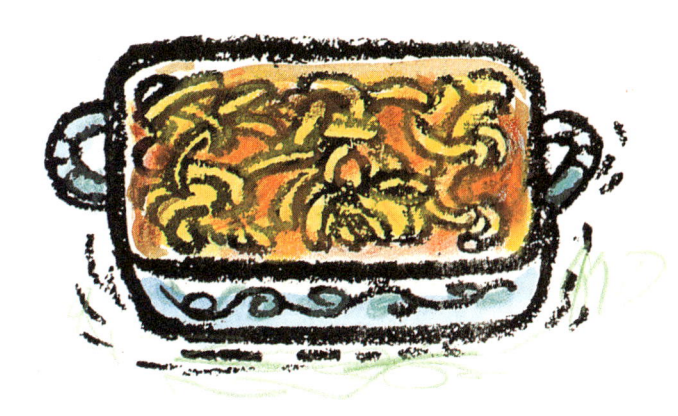

SPECIAL DIETS

Calories per SV	Protein g/ SV	Full-Liquid	Soft	Fiber-Restricted	Low-Lactose
275	11			**	*

* Substitute formula for milk, use nondairy margarine and aged cheddar cheese.
** Each serving counts as 1 1/4 cups of milk.

Quickly prepared, this casserole may disappear just as fast at the table!

Cheesy Hamburger Casserole

1 cup macaroni, uncooked
1/2 lb. ground meat (beef, veal)
1/2 small onion, chopped
3/4 cup tomato sauce or chopped tomatoes
1/2 can (10 oz.) cheddar cheese soup

Cook macaroni until slightly tender. Drain, set aside. Brown ground meat and onions in small skillet. Add tomatoes and simmer 10 minutes. Oil a 1-quart casserole, and spoon in 1/3 of meat mixture. Add cooked macaroni, then the remainder of meat mixture. Spread cheese soup over all (may be frozen unbaked). Cover the casserole tightly and bake at 400° until bubbly. Serves 4.

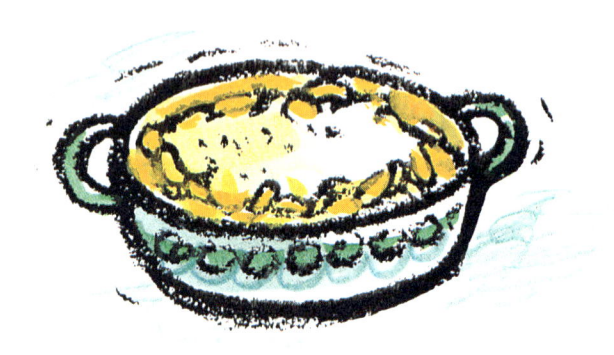

SPECIAL DIETS

Calories per SV	Protein g/ SV	Full-Liquid	Soft	Fiber-Restricted	Low-Lactose
215	16				*

* Omit cheese soup, add 1/2 cup water and 2 ozs. aged cheddar cheese.

This is a simple one-dish meal, a cousin to Quiche Lorraine. It is just the thing needed for a night when you don't want to fuss.

Cheese-Spinach Pie

1/3 cup chopped onion
1 tbsp. margarine
1/4 lb. sliced cheese
   (Swiss or Muenster)
1 cup cooked, chopped spinach
   (drained)

3 large eggs
1/3-1/2 cup of milk
1/2 tsp. salt
dash pepper
9-inch pie shell

Cook onion in margarine until tender; cool. Lay slices of cheese over pie dough, follow with spinach, then onions. Beat eggs, adding enough milk to make 1 cup. Add seasonings and pour over ingredients in the pie shell. Bake in 400° oven about 35 minutes, or until a knife comes out clean. Serve piping hot. (Can be frozen after baking.) Serves 4.

Variation: Substitute cooked, chopped broccoli, green beans, zucchini, or peas for spinach.

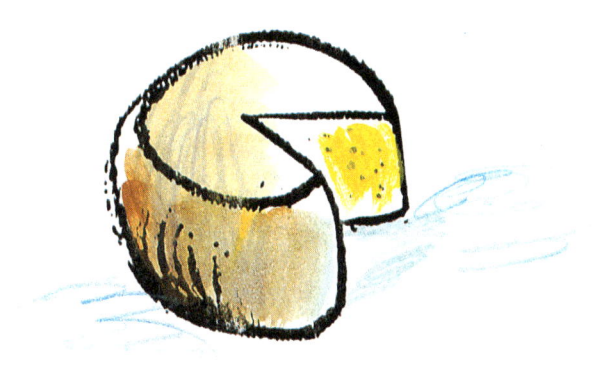

SPECIAL DIETS

Calories per SV	Protein g/ SV	Full-Liquid	Soft	Fiber-Restricted	Low-Lactose
454	18				*

* Substitute soy formula for milk. Use nondairy margarine and aged natural cheese and milk-free dough.

Here is a reliable, mildly flavored recipe which can be adapted to your needs.

Basic Meatloaf or Meatballs

2 tbsp. dry bread or cracker crumbs
1 tbsp. water
1/2 lb. ground beef or veal
1 egg

1/4 tsp. minced onion
salt and pepper to taste
1 tbsp. oil or margarine
2 slices onion

Combine crumbs and water in small mixing bowl. Add meat, minced onion, egg, and seasonings. Mix until well blended. Form into patties, 1-inch meatballs, or a loaf. Brown in oil or margarine in skillet, turn to brown both sides. Add sliced onion, lower heat, cover and simmer for at least 15 minutes, 30 minutes for meatloaf. You also can bake at 350°. For meatballs, bake 30 minutes, turning after 15 minutes. For meatloaf, bake 1 hour. Can be frozen raw or cooked. Serves 4.

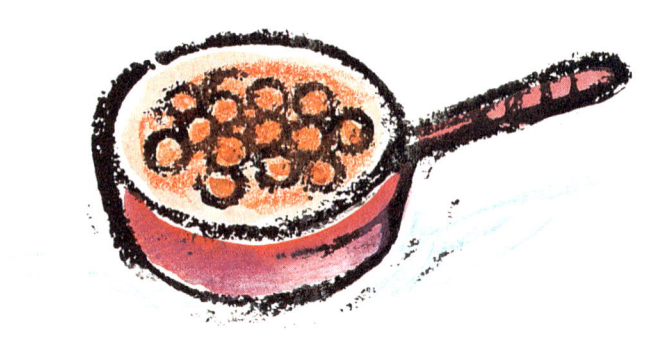

SPECIAL DIETS

Calories per SV	Protein g/ SV	Full-Liquid	Soft	Fiber-Restricted	Low-Lactose
125	13				*

* Use milk-free bread crumbs.

A favorite of young and old that is easy to eat.

Sloppy Joes

1/2 lb. ground meat
1 small onion, diced

1/2 cup quick barbecue sauce
 (see page 63)
1 tbsp. raw oatmeal

Brown meat and onion in skillet. Add barbecue sauce, oatmeal, and enough water to cover meat. Heat to boiling, turn down heat to simmer, cover pan, and cook 15 minutes or until thickened and meat is soft. Serve on buns, toast, or hard rolls. Can be frozen after cooking. Serves 4.

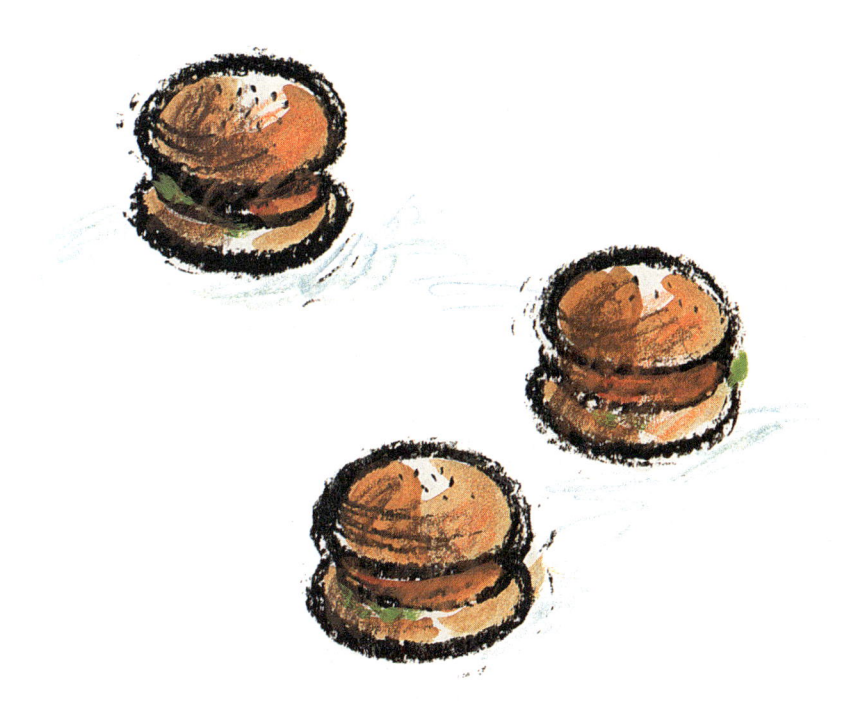

SPECIAL DIETS

Calories per SV	Protein g/ SV	Full-Liquid	Soft	Fiber-Restricted	Low-Lactose
160	12				

These are tender meatballs with gourmet flavor.

Swedish Meatballs

1 lb. ground round steak
½ cup plain bread crumbs
1 egg, slightly beaten
⅔ tsp. salt
dash pepper and allspice
1 tbsp. margarine

Mix all ingredients except margarine with a fork until well blended. Form into balls, brown in margarine in medium-sized skillet. Remove meatballs from pan. Make a thickened gravy with the drippings. Return meatballs to gravy and simmer, covered, for 1 to 1½ hours. May be frozen raw or cooked. Serves 4.

Contributed by D. Ruth Gilbert.

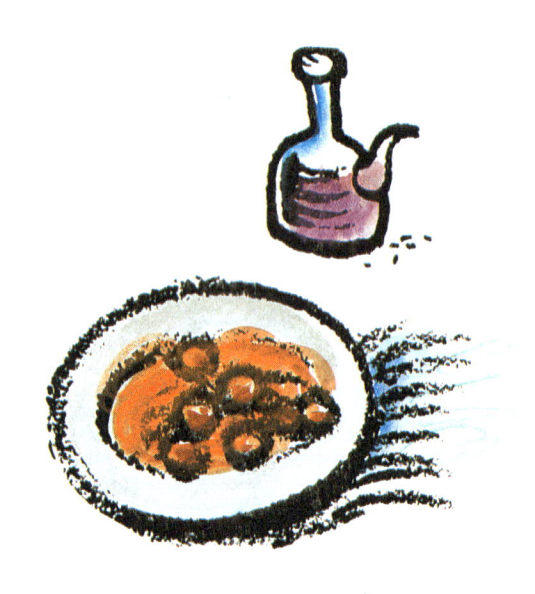

SPECIAL DIETS

Calories per SV	Protein g/ SV	Full-Liquid	Soft	Fiber-Restricted	Low-Lactose
281	25				*

* Use milk-free bread crumbs.

Supremely simple to make, this is a delightfully seasoned entrée.

Chicken Supreme

1 can (10 oz.) cream of
    mushroom soup
1/2 cup orange juice
1/2 cup water

1 cup rice, uncooked
6 pieces chicken
1/4 envelope onion soup mix

Combine first four ingredients and pour into greased 2-quart casserole. Lay chicken on top. Sprinkle with dry onion soup mix. Cover casserole, airtight, with heavy aluminum foil. Bake 2 hours without opening the foil, at 350°. Can be frozen after baking. Serves 6.

Contributed by a patient.

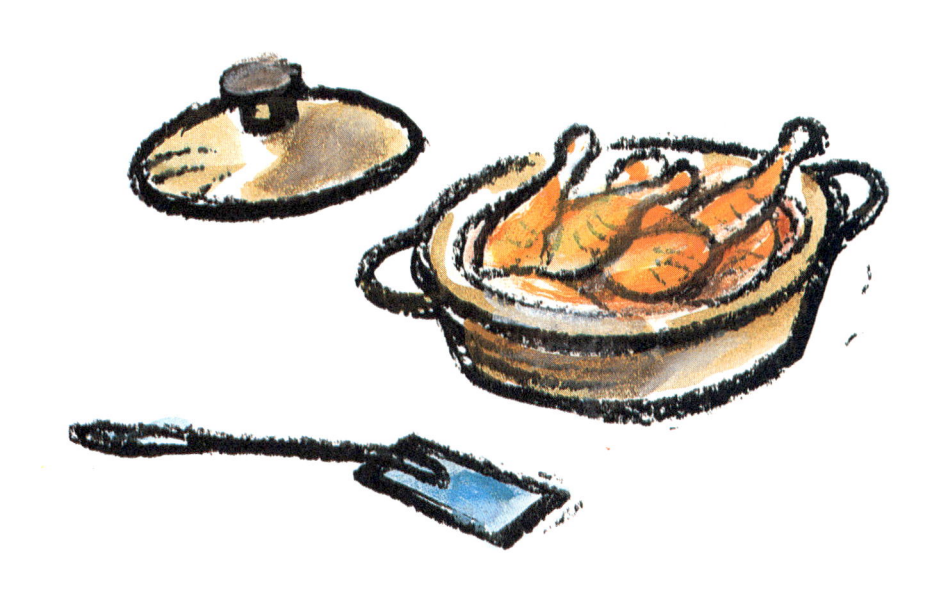

SPECIAL DIETS

Calories per SV	Protein g/ SV	Full-Liquid	Soft	Fiber-Restricted	Low-Lactose
295	18				

Tender and lightly seasoned, this simple dish can be a complete meal with rice, noodles, or mashed potatoes.

Chicken Skillet Supper

2-3 lbs. frying chicken, cut up
1/2 can (10 oz.) vegetarian-
   vegetable soup
1 can water
2 sprigs of parsley
1 basil leaf (optional)

Place chicken, skin side down, in cold skillet. Brown over medium heat, turning to brown inside. Remove from heat (chicken skin can easily be removed at this point). Pour off all fat remaining in skillet. Replace chicken, pour soup and water over chicken, and add seasonings. Simmer 1 hour in covered skillet, turning pieces once to keep them moist. May be frozen after cooking. Serves 4.

Tomato special: Substitute 1/2 can of cream of tomato for vegetarian-vegetable soup. Add 1 package (10 oz.) of mixed frozen vegetables with the soup and water.

Creamy chicken: Substitute 1/2 can of cream of chicken for vegetarian-vegetable soup, add 1 package (10 oz.) frozen peas and carrots.

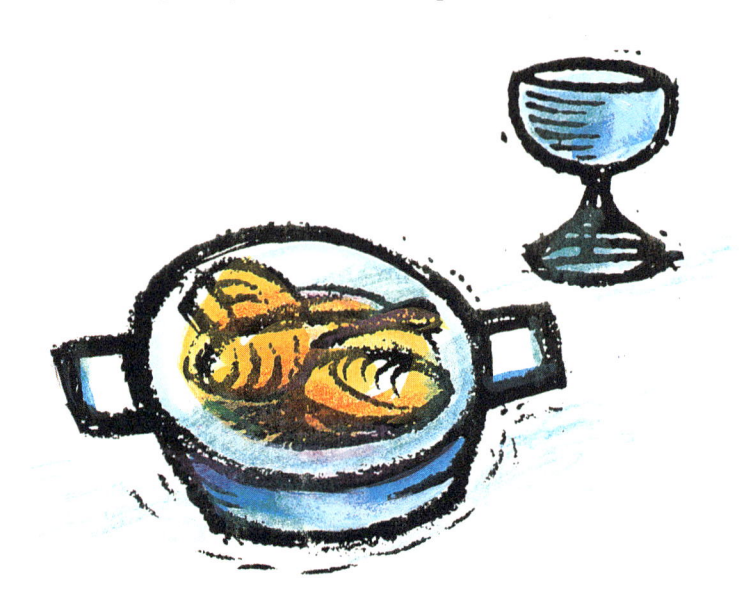

SPECIAL DIETS

Calories per SV	Protein g/ SV	Full-Liquid	Soft	Fiber-Restricted	Low-Lactose
200	24				

This mild-flavored tuna dish is complemented with a tossed salad.

Robert's Tuna Bake

1 can (7 oz.) water-packed tuna, broken into small pieces
1 can (10 oz.) tomato soup
½ cup milk
¼ lb. American or cheddar cheese
1 lb. box of elbow macaroni, cooked

Mix first four ingredients in saucepan and heat until cheese melts. Add macaroni to sauce and mix well. Pour into greased baking dish and bake at 350° for 20 minutes. Serves 8.

Chicken Noodle Bake: Substitute cream of celery soup for tomato, 1 cup diced chicken for tuna, cooked noodles for elbow macaroni.

Egg Noodle Bake: Substitute cream of chicken soup for tomato, 3 or more sliced hard-boiled eggs for tuna, and cooked noodles for elbow macaroni.

Contributed by Mr. Robert L. Card.

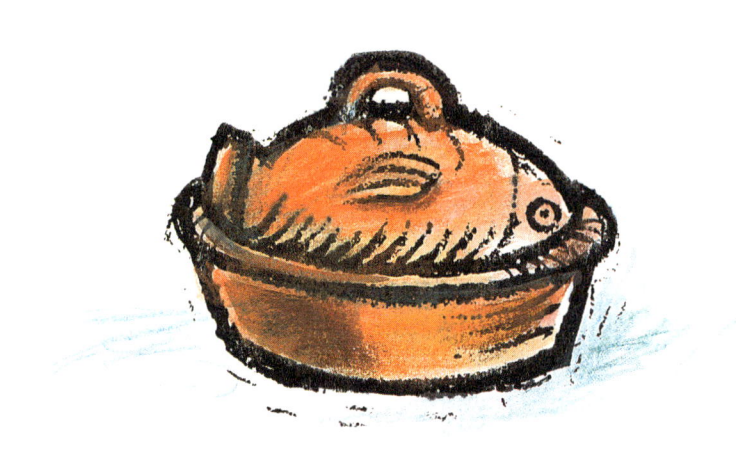

SPECIAL DIETS

Calories per SV	Protein g/ SV	Full-Liquid	Soft	Fiber-Restricted	Low-Lactose
435	24			**	*

* Substitute soy formula for milk. Use aged cheddar cheese.
** Each serving counts as ½ cup of milk.

A surprising balance of flavors will please busy cooks and their families.

Tuna Broccoli Casserole

2 packages (10 oz.) frozen broccoli, whole or chopped
2 cans (7 oz.) water-packed tuna broken into small pieces
1 can (10 oz.) cream of mushroom soup diluted with 1/2 cup of milk
1 cup grated cheddar or American cheese
1/2 cup plain bread crumbs
2 tbsp. melted margarine

Cook broccoli according to package directions, drain, and place in shallow 2-quart casserole. Add tuna and cover with diluted mushroom soup. Sprinkle with cheese. Add bread crumbs to melted butter and sprinkle over casserole. Bake at 350° for 20 minutes. Serves 5.

Contributed by a patient.

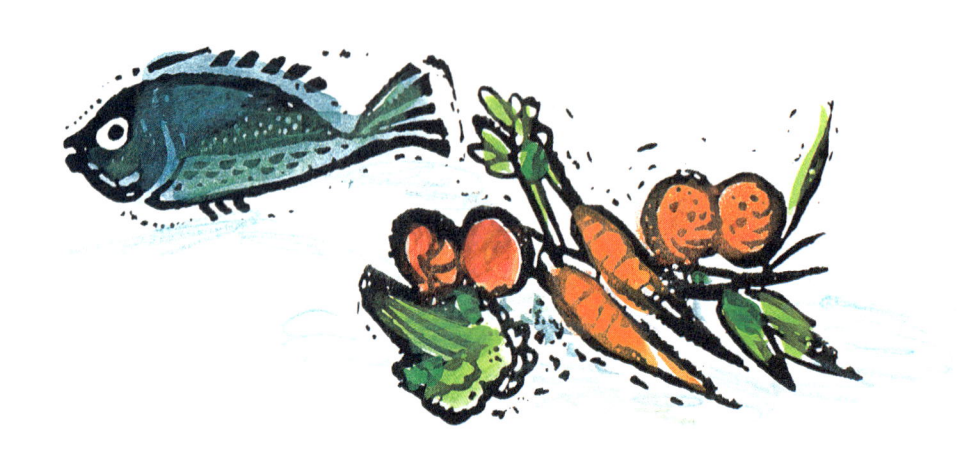

SPECIAL DIETS

Calories per SV	Protein g/ SV	Full-Liquid	Soft	Fiber-Restricted	Low-Lactose
290	25			**	*

* Substitute aged cheddar cheese, nondairy margarine, and use water instead of milk.
** Each serving counts as 3/4 cup of milk.

This light potato salad is mildly seasoned for the sensitive palate.

Creamy Potato Salad

1/3 cup plain low-fat yogurt
1/3 cup mayonnaise
1/4 tsp. finely minced or
　scraped onion
1 sprig of parsley, finely chopped

1/4 cup chopped celery or
　green pepper (optional)
2 potatoes, boiled and diced
2 hard-boiled eggs, diced
salt to taste

Blend yogurt, mayonnaise, onion, parsley, celery, and pepper. Stir in remaining ingredients. Cover and refrigerate for several hours. Serves 4.

Ricotta Potato Salad: Add 1/3 cup ricotta cheese to mayonnaise.

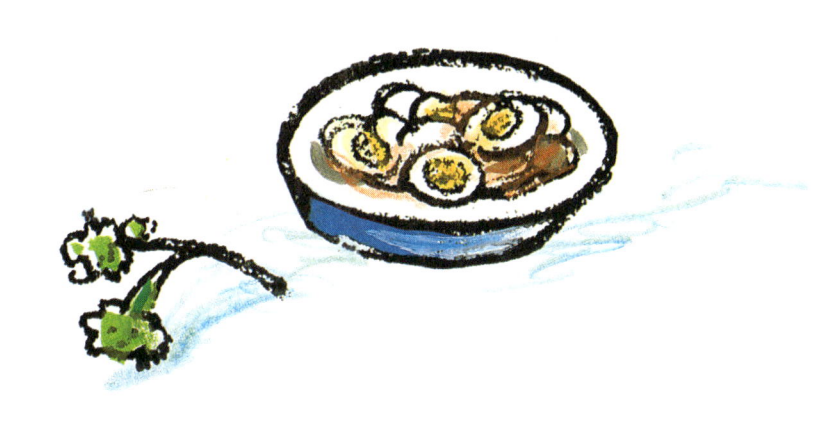

SPECIAL DIETS

Calories per SV	Protein g/ SV	Full-Liquid	Soft	Fiber-Restricted	Low-Lactose
245	5		**		*

* Use yogurt made only from cultured pasteurized milk.
** Omit onion, celery, green pepper.

This is a quick, flavorful sauce everybody can enjoy on eggs or meat.

Creole Sauce

1/2 small onion, sliced
1 or 2 frying peppers (1 bell pepper) cleaned and sliced
2 tbsp. oil
2 cups chopped fresh tomatoes or 1 can (15 oz.) tomatoes
1/2 tsp. salt
2 tbsp. sugar
1 tsp. vinegar
1 tbsp. cornstarch
water

Fry onion and peppers in oil until onion is clear and pepper is spotted with brown. Add tomatoes, salt, sugar, and vinegar. Bring to boiling, turn down to simmer. Cover and cook at least 20 minutes to blend the flavors. Thicken just before serving with cornstarch dissolved in a little water. Use on eggs or meat. Makes 2 cups. Serves 4.

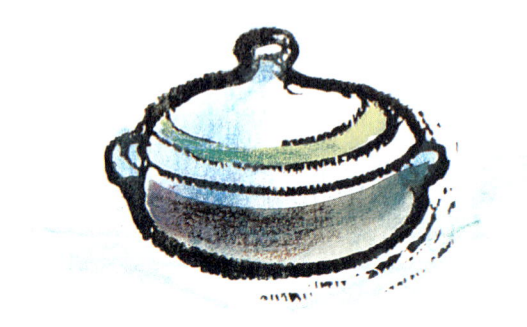

SPECIAL DIETS

Calories per SV	Protein g/ SV	Full-Liquid	Soft	Fiber-Restricted	Low-Lactose
150	2				

Use this sauce on hot dogs, chicken, or meatballs.

Quick Barbecue Sauce

1/2 cup catsup
2 tsps. salad style mustard
1/2 tsp. lemon juice

1 tbsp. brown sugar
1/2 tsp. onion salt

Mix together in small saucepan. Heat until boiling, stirring as it cooks.

Serving suggestions: Make Sloppy Joes. Use as a barbecue sauce for hot dogs, chicken, or meatballs. (It easily will coat eight pieces of chicken.) Use as a marinade for chicken or meat. Pour over pieces in a deep dish and refrigerate in marinade at least 12 hours to tenderize. Makes 1/2 cup.

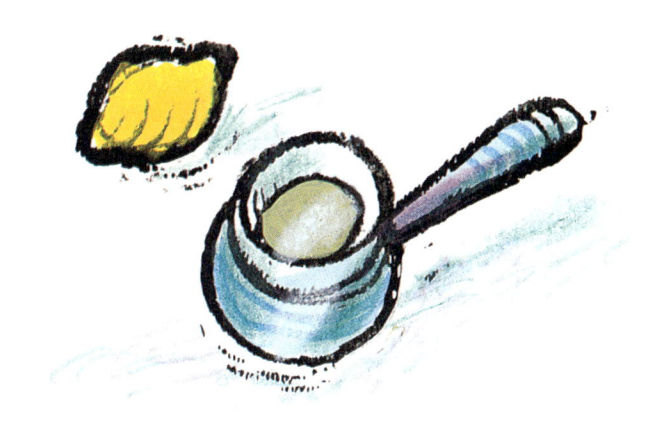

SPECIAL DIETS

Calories per SV	Protein g/ SV	Full-Liquid	Soft	Fiber-Restricted	Low-Lactose
208	2				

An unexpected favorite, this tangy sauce is often used on meat or chicken.

Sweet and Sour Sauce

1/4 cup vinegar
1 cup catsup
1 tbsp. soy sauce
1/2 red or green pepper, cubed
1/2 cup honey or brown sugar (packed)

1/2 tsp. salt
1 can (8 oz.) pineapple chunks (optional)
water
2 tbsp. cornstarch

Mix all ingredients except cornstarch in saucepan. Bring to boil. Turn heat down to simmer, stirring occasionally and cook for at least 20 minutes to allow flavors to blend. Dissolve cornstarch in small amount of water. Add, stirring until thickened. (You can omit cornstarch and allow the sauce to thicken by cooking it longer.) Use on meat or chicken. Makes 2 cups.

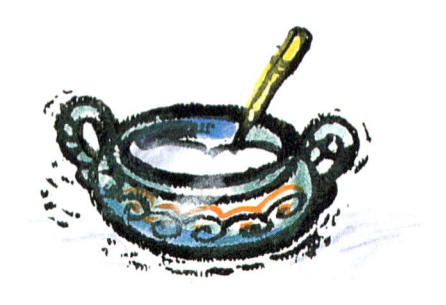

SPECIAL DIETS

Calories per SV	Protein g/ SV	Full-Liquid	Soft	Fiber-Restricted	Low-Lactose
590	3				

These pancakes have double the protein of regular pancakes. Two of them equal 1 ounce of meat in protein content.

High-Protein Pancakes

1/2 cup milk
2 tbsp. dry milk
1 egg (2 for a thinner, crepe-type)

2 tsps. of oil
1/2-3/4 cups pancake mix

Measure milk, dry milk, egg, and oil into blender or bowl. Beat until egg is well blended. Add pancake mix. Stir or blend at low speed until mix is wet but some lumps remain. Cook on hot, greased griddle or frying pan. Turn when firm to brown the other side. These can be kept warm in a warm oven or in a covered pan on low heat. Makes seven 4" pancakes.

Note: If there is batter left over, it will keep 1 day in the refrigerator, or it can be made into pancakes, cooled, and wrapped in foil to be frozen for later use. To reheat, leave in foil and place in 450° oven for 15 minutes. If using a toaster oven, unwrap them, brush with margarine, and toast as for light toast.

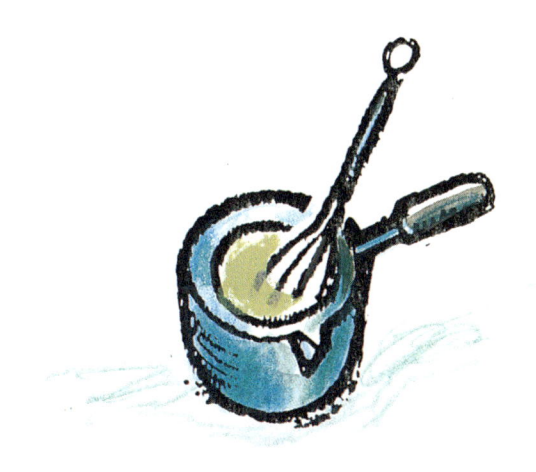

SPECIAL DIETS

Calories per SV	Protein g/ SV	Full-Liquid	Soft	Fiber-Restricted	Low-Lactose
77	3			*	

* The dry and fluid milk in the entire recipe count as 1 cup of milk.

These pancakes have the high protein quality without a drop of milk.

Low-Lactose Pancakes

1 egg (2 for crepe-type)
1/2 cup soy formula

2 tsps. milk-free margarine, melted
1/2 cup milk-free pancake mix

Put egg, soy formula, and melted margarine into bowl or blender. Beat to blend. Stir in mix until wet but some lumps remain. Cook on greased or oiled pan (use only milk-free margarine, bacon fat, or shortening) until firm enough to turn over. Brown other side. Keep warm in oven or covered pan on low heat. If you wish to freeze pancakes, follow directions in recipe for High-Protein Pancakes. Makes six 4" pancakes.

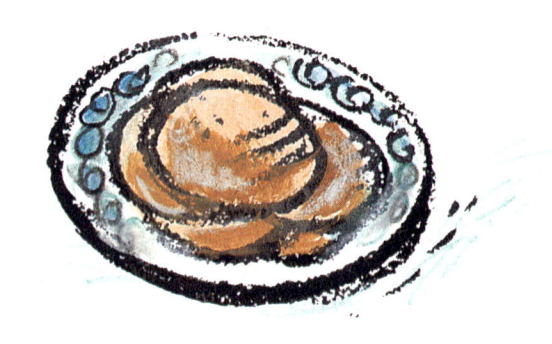

SPECIAL DIETS

Calories per SV	Protein g/ SV	Full-Liquid	Soft	Fiber-Restricted	Low-Lactose
88	2				

This doubles the protein in each cup of milk.

Fortified Milk

1 quart milk, homogenized or
   1% low-fat

1 cup instant nonfat dry milk

Pour liquid milk into deep bowl. Add dry milk and beat slowly with beater until dry milk is dissolved (usually less than 5 minutes). Refrigerate. The flavor improves after several hours. Makes 1 quart.

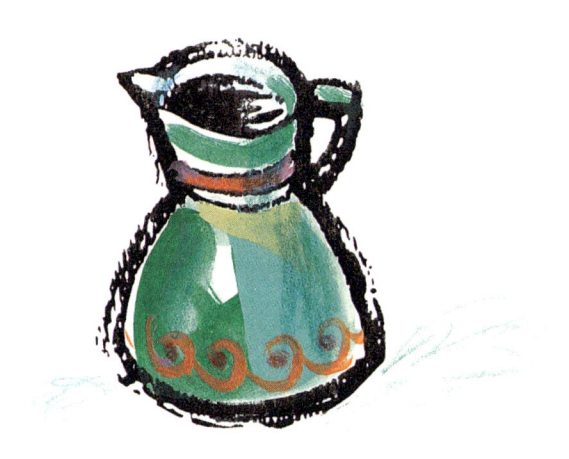

			SPECIAL DIETS		
Calories per SV	Protein g/ SV	Full-Liquid	Soft	Fiber-Restricted	Low-Lactose

WHOLE MILK

275	19				

1% MILK

195	19				

A tasty banana shake is a rich potassium source.

Vera's Banana Milkshake

1 whole ripe banana, sliced
1 cup milk
vanilla (few drops)

Measure into blender and blend at high speed until smooth. Serves 1.
Banana-Butterscotch: Add 2 tbsp. of butterscotch sauce with banana.
Contributed by Vera Bagley.

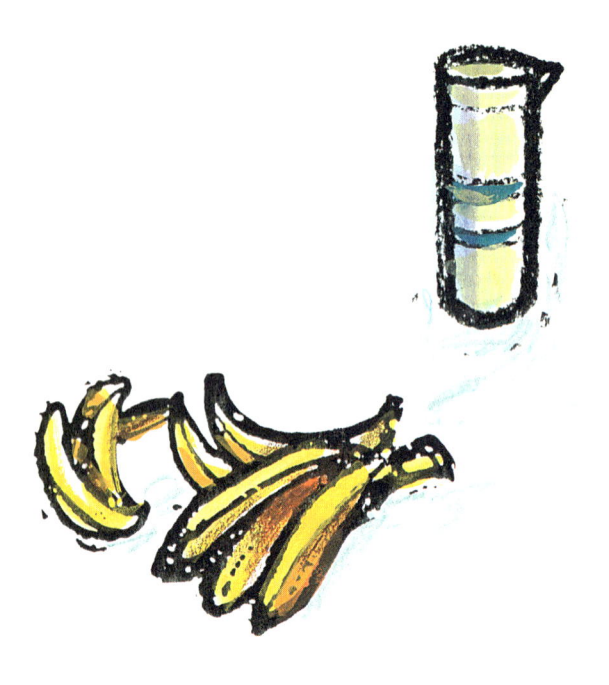

SPECIAL DIETS

Calories per SV	Protein g/ SV	Full-Liquid	Soft	Fiber-Restricted	Low-Lactose
275	9			**	*

* Substitute soy formula for milk.
** One milkshake counts as 1 cup of a daily 2-cup milk allowance.

This drink has the flavor of fresh strawberries, but comes from the freezer.

Pearl's Strawberry Milkshake

1/2 cup frozen strawberries
1 scoop ice cream
1/2 cup milk

Mix or blend until smooth. Serves 1.

Contributed by Pearl L. Howard.

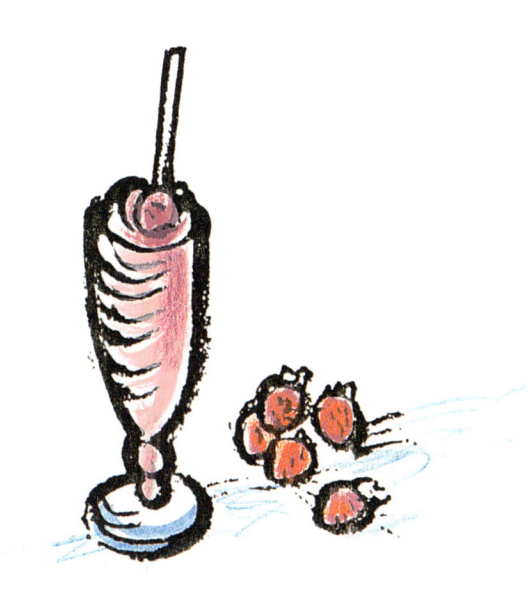

SPECIAL DIETS

Calories per SV	Protein g/ SV	Full-Liquid	Soft	Fiber-Restricted	Low-Lactose
355	7			*	

* Count as 1 cup of a daily 2-cup milk allowance.

These favorite milkshake flavors have extra protein.

High-Protein Milkshakes

1 cup fortified milk
1 generous scoop ice cream
1/2 tsp. vanilla

2 tbsp. of butterscotch, chocolate, or your favorite fruit syrup or sauce

Measure all ingredients into blender. Blend at low speed for about 10 seconds. Serves 1.

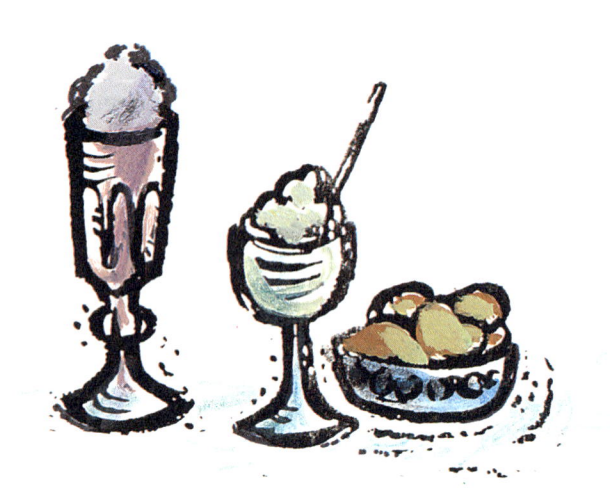

SPECIAL DIETS

Calories per SV	Protein g/ SV	Full-Liquid	Soft	Fiber-Restricted	Low-Lactose
485	22				

Make imitation milkshakes for people who cannot drink milk or eat ice cream. Enjoy! Enjoy!

Citrus Fake Shakes

1 frozen citrus fruit juice bar (2 1/2 oz.) or 2 bars (1 3/4 oz.) same flavor
1/2 cup chilled soy-based milk substitute/nutritional supplement
1/4 tsp. vanilla

Remove citrus bar from freezer and allow to thaw slightly (about 5-10 minutes until soft). Break bar into pieces into blender. Add other ingredients and blend at low speed for 10 seconds. Serves 1.

Double Citrus: Add 1 tbsp. frozen orange juice concentrate and 1 tbsp. sugar to the lemon or orange flavor Fake Shake before blending. This version has 192 calories and 3 grams of protein per cup.

Other Fake Shakes

Butterscotch

1/2 cup chilled or partially frozen soy-based milk substitute/
   nutritional supplement
1/4 tsp. vanilla
2 tbsp. milk-free butterscotch sauce

Blend all at low speed about 10 seconds. Using the partially frozen liquid will produce a much colder, thicker shake. Serves 1.

Chocolate

Use 2 tbsp. chocolate syrup in place of butterscotch.
(Commercial chocolate syrups are often made without milk or lactose; always read the ingredient labels.)

Butterscotch-Banana

Add 1/2 well ripened, sliced banana to ingredients for butterscotch shake.

Peanut Butter-Honey

Omit butterscotch sauce. Mix together in a cup: 1/4 cup soy formula or nondairy creamer, 2 tbsp. smooth peanut butter, 1 tbsp. honey, and 1/4 tsp. vanilla. Place partially frozen liquid in blender, then add peanut butter mixture. Blend for about 10 seconds or until smooth.

Fake Shake Sherbet

Follow recipe for Peanut Butter-Honey (you can double or triple recipe). Pour shake into small container. Freeze 2 hours or until it begins to harden around edges. Scrape into bowl and mix thoroughly, until lumps disappear. Return to container and refreeze 2 hours or until firm.

Other Frozen Fake Shakes

The Butterscotch, Chocolate, or Butterscotch-Banana shakes (on page 71) can be frozen using the same method as for Fake Shake Sherbert.

Instant Breakfast Shake

1 package instant breakfast mix
1 cup whole milk
1/4 cup instant nonfat dry milk
1 cup ice cream (2 to 3 scoops)* (Sherbet may be substituted for ice cream.)
1 egg (poached or soft-boiled), if desired

Mix or blend until smooth. Add more milk for a thinner shake. If shake tastes too sweet, add a few drops of lemon juice. Serves 1.

Make-Your-Own Shake

You can add any of the following to the Instant Breakfast Shake recipe:
- 1/2 large banana
- 1 to 2 tbsp. chocolate sauce
- 1 tsp. instant coffee plus sugar to taste
- 1 tbsp. malted milk powder
- 1/2 cup canned fruit
- 1/2 tsp. vanilla flavoring plus 1/4 tsp. cinnamon
- 1 tbsp. molasses
- fresh or frozen fruit, as allowed

Try something not listed, or mix together to make new combinations, or ask the registered dietitian for suggestions.

Homemade Peanut Butter Shake

1 cup vanilla-flavored, soy-based, nutritional supplement
1 pint low-fat vanilla ice cream
1 cup water
1/4 cup ginger ale
1 banana
5 tbsp. peanut butter

Add all ingredients to a blender and mix thoroughly until smooth. Refrigerate unused portion. Serves 4.

*Each serving counts as 1/2 cup of a daily 2-cup milk allowance.

SPECIAL DIETS

	Calories per SV	Protein g/ SV	Full-Liquid	Soft	Fiber-Restricted	Low-Lactose
CITRUS	114	3				
BUTTERSCOTCH	222	3				*
CHOCOLATE	165	3				
BUTTERSCOTCH BANANA	274	3				*
PEANUT BUTTER-HONEY	255	13				
FAKE SHAKE SHERBET	255	13				
INSTANT BREAKFAST SHAKE (WITHOUT EGG)	640	24				
INSTANT BREAKFAST SHAKE (WITH EGG)	715	31				
HOMEMADE PEANUT BUTTER SHAKE	285	9			*	

*Each serving counts as 1/2 cup of a daily 2-cup milk allowance.

It is important to know whether your physician allows alcohol before you sample the enriched drinks.

Fruit Smoothie

2 tbsp. blackberry or cherry cordial
3/4 cup chilled or partially frozen
    half-and-half

Mix or blend until smooth. Serve in a fancy glass, frosted if you like. Serves 1.

Panamanian Smoothie
Omit cordial; add 2 tbsp. chocolate syrup and 2 tbsp. rum.

Creme de Menthe Smoothie
Omit cordial; add 2 tbsp. creme de menthe and 2 tbsp. vanilla ice cream (omit ice cream for low-lactose).

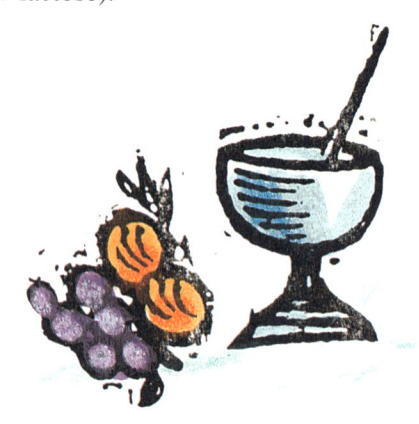

SPECIAL DIETS

	Calories per SV	Protein g/ SV	Full-Liquid	Soft	Fiber-Restricted	Low-Lactose
FRUIT	295	5			**	*
PANAMANIAN	400	6			**	*
CREME DE MENTHE	330	6			**	*

* Substitute nondairy creamer for half-and-half; omit ice cream.
** Each serving containing half-and-half counts as 3/4 cup milk; count 2 tbsp. of ice cream toward the daily 2-cup milk allowance.

An occasional drink has helped boost many a lagging appetite.

Amaretto Creme

1/2 cup chilled half-and-half
2 tbsp. vanilla ice cream
1 tbsp. Amaretto cordial

Mix until smooth. Serve in stemmed glass. Serves 1.

Butterscotch Brandy Creme
Omit Amaretto; add 2 tbsp. butterscotch sauce and 1 tbsp. brandy.

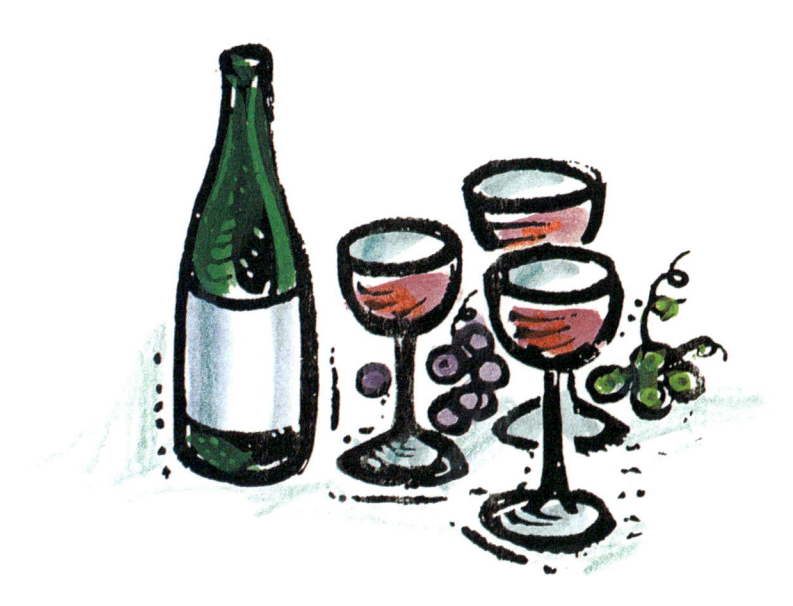

SPECIAL DIETS

Calories per SV	Protein g/ SV	Full-Liquid	Soft	Fiber-Restricted	Low-Lactose
245	4			**	*

* Substitute nondairy creamer and omit ice cream (Amaretto).
  Substitute nondairy creamer and milk-free butterscotch sauce (Butterscotch Brandy Creme).
** Each serving counts as 1/2 cup milk.

The sweet-tart taste of this sauce is a change from sweet syrup. It is good on pancakes and waffles.

Fresh Peach Sauce

1 large peach, peeled and thinly sliced
1 1/2 tbsp. sugar

1/4 cup water
1 tsp. cornstarch
dash nutmeg

Combine ingredients in a small pan, stir until cornstarch is dissolved. Cook over medium heat until sauce boils and is thickened. Serves 1.

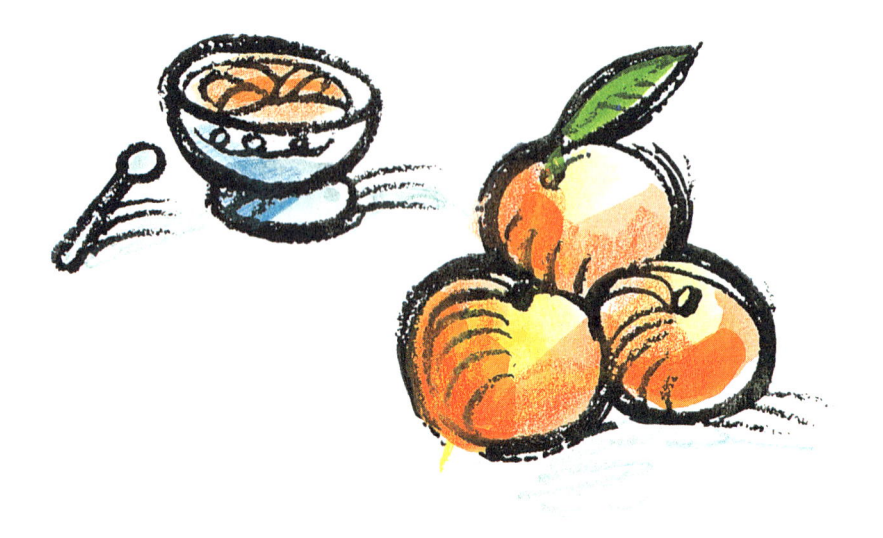

SPECIAL DIETS

Calories per SV	Protein g/ SV	Full-Liquid	Soft	Fiber-Restricted	Low-Lactose
140	0				

This tasty sauce is good for many toppings.

Milk-Free Butterscotch Sauce

1/2 cup brown sugar, packed
2 tsp. cornstarch
1/4 cup nondairy creamer
1/4 cup water

1 tbsp. honey
1 tbsp. milk-free margarine
1/2 tsp. vanilla

Mix brown sugar and cornstarch in small saucepan. Slowly add nondairy creamer and water, stirring until cornstarch dissolves. Add honey and margarine. Cook over medium heat, stirring constantly, until sauce is thickened and comes to a boil. Remove from heat. Add vanilla. Cook and store in a covered container in refrigerator. Makes about 1/2 cup.

Milk-Free Chocolate: Stir in 1 heaping tbsp. cocoa with cornstarch. If too thick, add a little water after it comes to a boil.

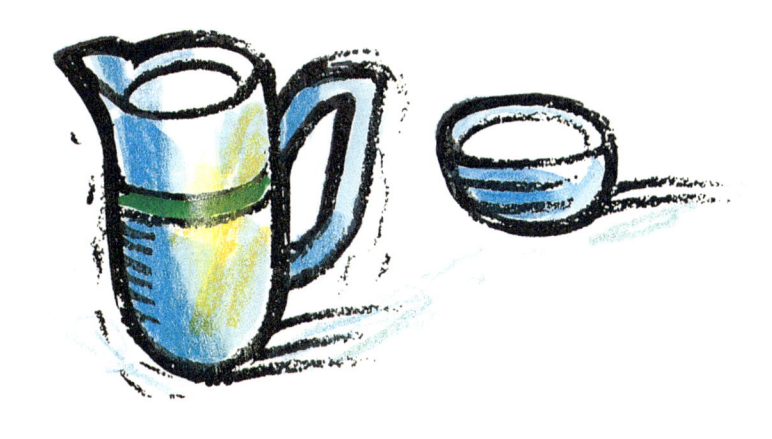

SPECIAL DIETS

Calories per SV	Protein g/ SV	Full-Liquid	Soft	Fiber-Restricted	Low-Lactose
85	0				

This is a high-protein snack of good quality.

Peanut Butter Snack Spread

1 tbsp. instant dry milk
1 tsp. water
1 tsp. vanilla

1 tbsp. honey
3 heaping tbsp. creamy peanut butter

Combine dry milk, water, and vanilla, stirring to moisten. Add honey and peanut butter, stirring slowly until liquid begins to blend with peanut butter. Spread between graham crackers or milk lunch crackers. The spread can also be formed into balls, chilled, and eaten as candy. Keeps well in refrigerator but is difficult to spread when cold. Makes 1/3 cup.

Molasses Taffy Flavor: Substitute molasses for honey.

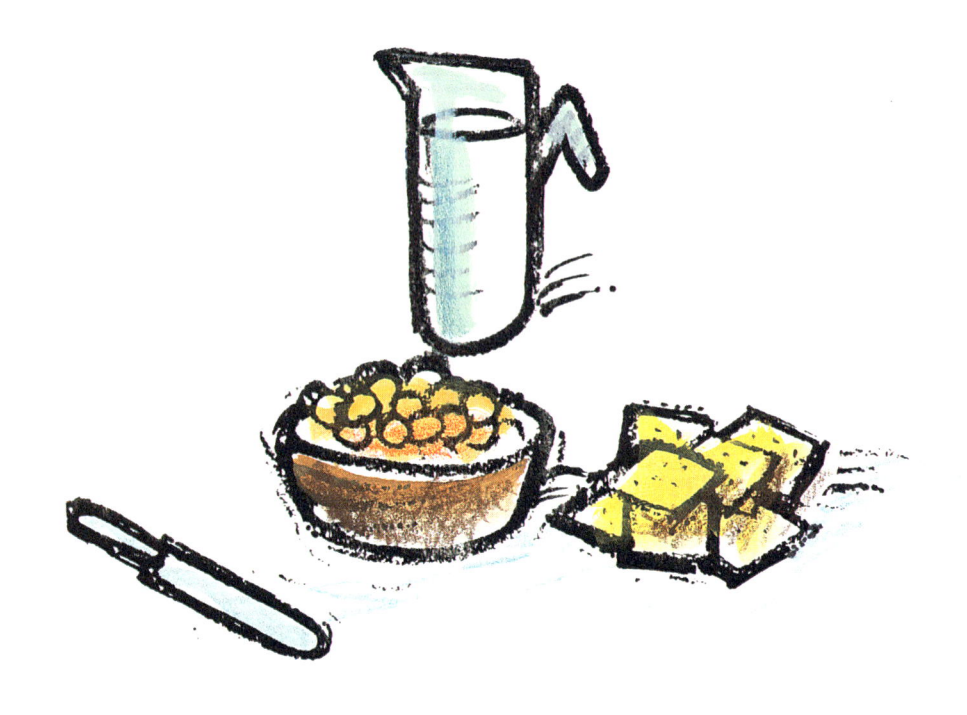

SPECIAL DIETS

Calories per SV	Protein g/ SV	Full-Liquid	Soft	Fiber-Restricted	Low-Lactose
440	17			**	*

* Substitute 1 tbsp. soy formula for milk and water.
** Count dry milk as 1/4 cup milk of a daily 2-cups milk allowance.

Here is a natural fiber snack or cereal.

Granola I

1 1/2 cups quick oatmeal
1/2 cup regular wheat germ
1/2 cup coconut
1/2 tsp. salt

1/2 cup chopped nuts
2 tbsp. oil
2/3 cup sweetened condensed milk

Measure oatmeal, wheat germ, coconut, salt, and nuts into mixing bowl, stirring to blend. Add oil and mix thoroughly. Pour in condensed milk and blend well. Sprinkle a handful of wheat germ on a cookie sheet and gently spread mixture on top. Bake in 325° oven about 25 minutes. Check mix as it bakes—after the first 10 minutes, mix will begin to brown. Stir it on cookie sheet every 10 minutes until it is as brown as you like. Cool on pan; store in covered container in refrigerator.

Granola II: Omit milk. Add 1/2 cup honey. Bake as above.

Chocolate chip: Put hot mixture in bowl. Stir in 1/2 cup of chocolate chips.

Raisin: Stir in 1 cup of raisins after the mixture cools.

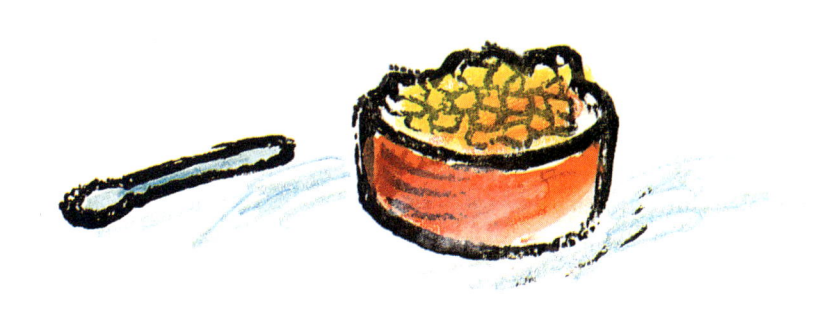

SPECIAL DIETS

Calories per SV	Protein g/ SV	Full-Liquid	Soft	Fiber-Restricted	Low-Lactose
GRANOLA I					
330	9				
GRANOLA II					
340	7				

Try a chewy, delightful bar, great with tea or for a snack for the children with milk.

Granola Bars

3/4 cup quick cooking oatmeal
1/2 cup Granola II (page 79)
1/2 cup coconut
1/2 cup brown sugar (packed)
1/4 cup melted margarine

1 egg
1/4 tsp. vanilla extract
1 tbsp. honey
1/4 tsp. salt
1/4 cup flour

Measure oatmeal, granola, coconut, and brown sugar together in deep bowl. Mix well. Pour melted margarine over all and blend thoroughly. Beat the egg, extract, honey, and salt together. Pour this over dry ingredients, stirring to blend. Add flour, stirring until smoothly mixed. Press mixture onto greased, floured 11x7-inch shallow baking pan or cookie sheet. Bake at 325° for 35 minutes. Cool slightly, cut into bars, and remove from the pan while warm. Makes 18 bars.

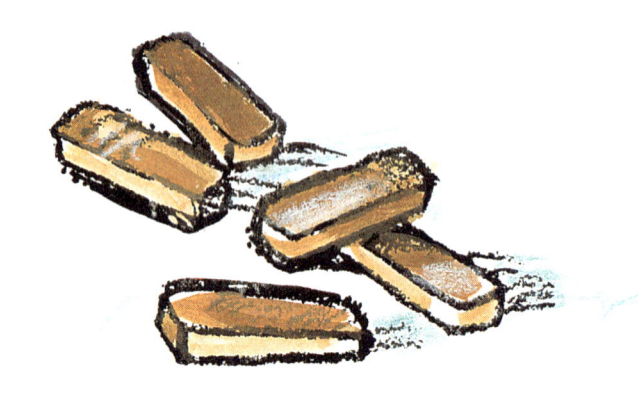

SPECIAL DIETS

Calories per SV	Protein g/ SV	Full-Liquid	Soft	Fiber-Restricted	Low-Lactose
60	2				

This soft, delightful dessert is made with bread and tasty apples.

Apple Brown Betty

4 cups thinly sliced pared apples or
   1 can (16 oz.) pie apples, drained
2 cups bread cubes or
   torn bread pieces

1/2 cup brown sugar, packed
1/8 tsp. ground cinnamon
2 tbsp. margarine
1/4 cup hot water

Grease 1-quart baking dish. Arrange half of apples on bottom of dish. Follow with half of bread, then half of sugar. Repeat layers. Sprinkle cinnamon over top, cut margarine in pieces and lay them on top, finish by pouring hot water over all. Cover and bake at 350° for 30 minutes, uncover and bake 10 minutes longer. Serve warm or chilled. Serves 4.

Apple Cheese Betty: Spoon 1 cup ricotta cheese over first layer of apples, bread, and sugar. Complete as above.

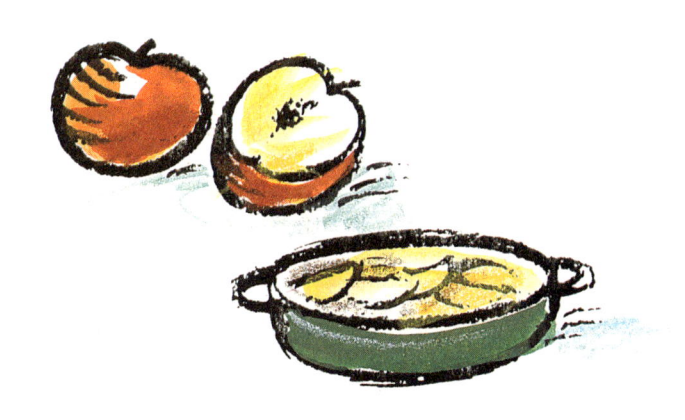

SPECIAL DIETS

Calories per SV	Protein g/ SV	Full-Liquid	Soft	Fiber-Restricted	Low-Lactose
WITHOUT CHEESE					
291	1			*	
WITH CHEESE					
342	4			**	

* Count apples as 2 servings fruit (maximum allowed per day).
** Count apples as above; also, each serving counts as 1 cup of a daily 2-cup milk allowance.

Delightful as a plain moist cake, this dessert is mouth-watering when iced with Helen's chocolate frosting (see page 85).

Adair's Apple Raisin Cake

1 3/4 cup coarsely chopped apples, or drained canned pie apples, chopped
3/4 cup brown sugar, packed
1/2 cup oil
1 egg, beaten
1/2 tsp. baking soda
1 tsp. baking powder
1/2 tsp. salt
1 1/2 cups flour
1 tsp. cinnamon
1/2 tsp. nutmeg
1/2 cup raisins, soaked in warm water until plump, then drained
1/2 cup chopped nuts

Measure apples and brown sugar into bowl. Add oil and eggs. Add dry ingredients and mix well. This dough will be stiff.

Add raisins and nuts. Stir to blend. Spread in 8-inch square pan. Bake at 350° for 40 minutes or until top springs back when touched. May be frozen. Serves 16.

Contributed by Adair Luciani.

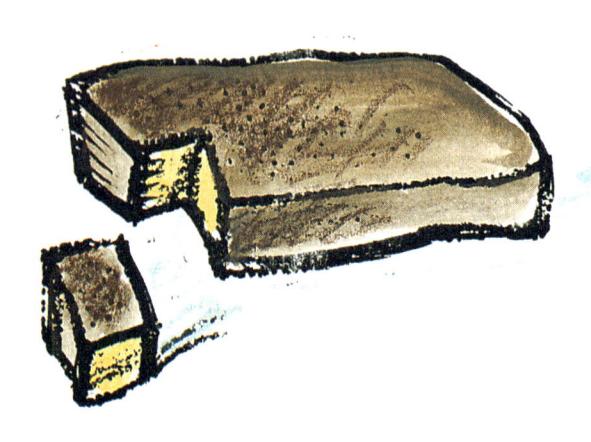

SPECIAL DIETS

Calories per SV	Protein g/ SV	Full-Liquid	Soft	Fiber-Restricted	Low-Lactose
200	3				

A speedy cheesecake is great for the single person.

Individual Cheese Pies

1 tbsp. ricotta cheese
1 tbsp. applesauce (pureed), peaches, or drained crushed pineapple

2 tsp. sugar
sprinkle of cinnamon
one 3-inch sugar cookie (store-bought)

Blend cheese, fruit, sugar, and cinnamon. Spoon over a sugar cookie, turned upside down so the sugar side is on the bottom next to the cookie sheet or foil. Bake at 350° for 15 minutes (the cookie softens as it absorbs the liquid from the fruit-cheese mixture; for a softer treat, lower the oven to 325°). Serves 1.

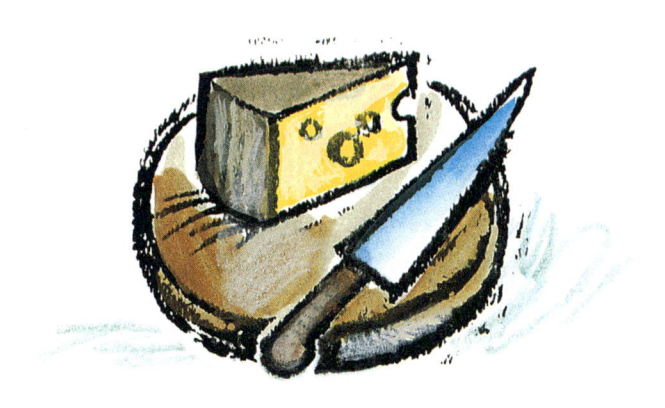

SPECIAL DIETS

Calories per SV	Protein g/ SV	Full-Liquid	Soft	Fiber-Restricted	Low-Lactose
85	2			*	

* Cheese is one-eighth of the 2-cup daily milk allowance.

This quickly made bread is high on the list of nourishing foods.

Banana-Nut Bread

2 eggs
3 medium well-ripened
   bananas, cut into chunks
1/4 cup of milk
1/4 cup of oil
1 tsp. vanilla extract
2 cups all-purpose flour
3/4 cup sugar
1 tbsp. baking powder
1/2 tsp. baking soda
1/2 tsp. salt
1/4 tsp. nutmeg
1/2-1 cup chopped walnuts or pecans,
   or wheat germ

Blend eggs, bananas, milk, oil, and vanilla at medium speed until smooth, about 15 seconds. Measure rest of ingredients into bowl and stir to mix. Make a well in the center of the dry ingredients and pour in banana mixture. Mix just enough to moisten. Add nuts. Spread batter into well greased 9x5x3-inch loaf pan or three small 5x3x2-inch pans. Bake the bread at 350°, about 1 hour for the large loaf and 35-45 minutes for the smaller ones. Makes 1 large loaf or 3 small loaves. Serves 16.

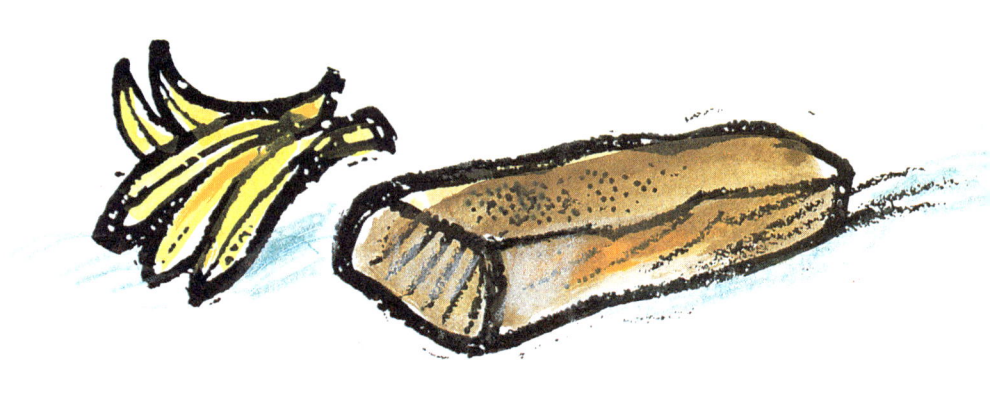

SPECIAL DIETS

Calories per SV	Protein g/ SV	Full-Liquid	Soft	Fiber-Restricted	Low-Lactose
185	3				*

* Omit milk, use nondairy creamer or soy formula.

Here is a good, fast-cooked icing.

Helen's Soft Chocolate Frosting

½ cup white sugar
½ cup brown sugar
3 heaping tbsp. cocoa

3 heaping tbsp. cornstarch
1 cup milk
3 tbsp. margarine

Mix first four ingredients together in saucepan until well blended. Gradually add milk. Add margarine. Cook over medium heat, stirring constantly until thick and smooth. (You may need to remove from heat occasionally to prevent sticking or lumping.) Ice cake while the frosting is still warm. Ices two 9-inch layers. Recipe can easily be cut in half for a single layer cake or cupcakes.

Contributed by Helen Monahan.

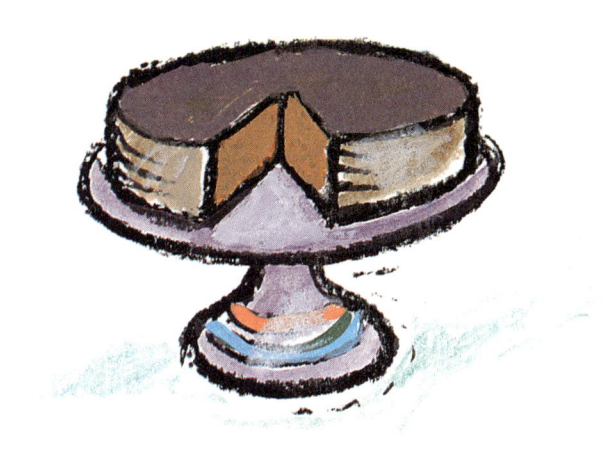

SPECIAL DIETS

Calories per SV	Protein g/ SV	Full-Liquid	Soft	Fiber-Restricted	Low-Lactose
91	1				*

* Substitute water for milk. Use nondairy margarine.

Fiber and nutrition are "partners" in these crunchy butterscotch cookies.

Cowboy Cookies

1 cup soft shortening or margarine
3/4 cup brown sugar, packed
3/4 cup granulated sugar
2 eggs
1 tsp. vanilla extract
2 cups flour
1/2 tsp. baking soda
1/2 tsp. salt
1 1/2 cups quick cooking oatmeal
1/2 cup coarsely chopped nuts or wheat germ
6 oz. chocolate chips
1 cup raisins

Cream shortening, add sugars, and beat well. Add the eggs and vanilla and stir to blend well. Add the dry ingredients at one time. Mix to blend thoroughly. Last, stir in oatmeal, nuts, chocolate chips, and raisins. Mix well. Drop by spoonfuls on cookie sheet and bake for 13-15 minutes in 350° oven. This dough freezes well and can be sliced later to make fresh cookies. Makes 4 dozen large cookies.

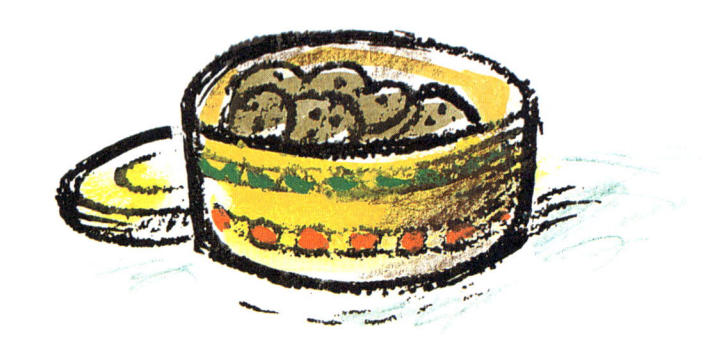

SPECIAL DIETS

Calories per SV	Protein g/ SV	Full-Liquid	Soft	Fiber-Restricted	Low-Lactose
135	2				

Peanut butter fans will like this nourishing bar cookie.

Peanut Butter Bars

1/4 cup margarine
1/4 cup smooth peanut butter
1 1/3 cups brown sugar, packed
2 eggs

1 1/2 cups flour
1 1/2 tsp. baking powder
1/2 cup chocolate chips
1/2 cup finely chopped nuts (optional)

Cream margarine and peanut butter. Add brown sugar and mix well. Add both eggs and mix until well blended. Stir in dry ingredients until blended, then chocolate chips and nuts. Spread batter in greased and floured 9-inch square pan. Bake at 350° for 30-35 minutes. Cool in pan. Cut when cooled into 36 bars.

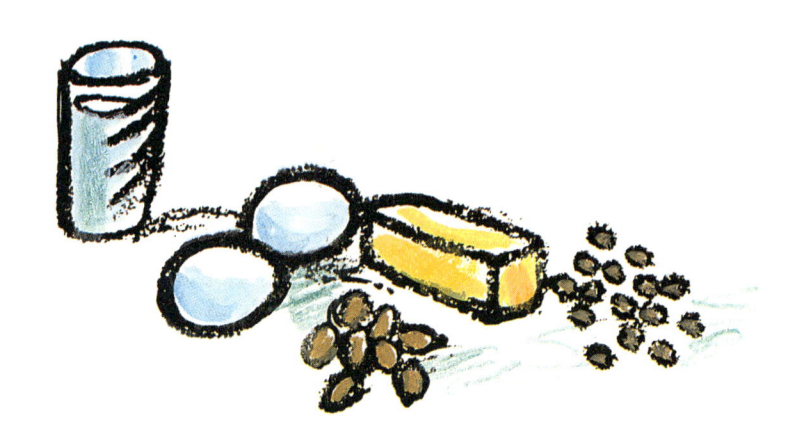

SPECIAL DIETS

Calories per SV	Protein g/ SV	Full-Liquid	Soft	Fiber-Restricted	Low-Lactose
90	2		*		

* Omit nuts.

Gelatin is a great way to enjoy fruit.

Fluffy Fruit Gelatin

1 cup cooked or canned peaches with syrup

1 package red gelatin (3 oz.)
1 cup boiling water

Blend fruit with syrup at high speed until smooth. Pour puréed fruit back into measuring cup and add enough syrup or water to make one cup. Dissolve gelatin in boiling water, pour into a bowl (deep enough to whip gelatin later). Stir in fruit purée. Cool. Refrigerate gelatin mixture until it piles softly, but is not firm. With cold beaters, whip the gelatin until foamy and doubled in volume. Refrigerate until firm. Serves 6.

Other fruits: Use pears, applesauce, or apricots in place of peaches.

Fluffy Fruit Cream: Fold in 1 cup of whipped cream or nondairy whipped toppings after whipping the gelatin. Refrigerate until firm.

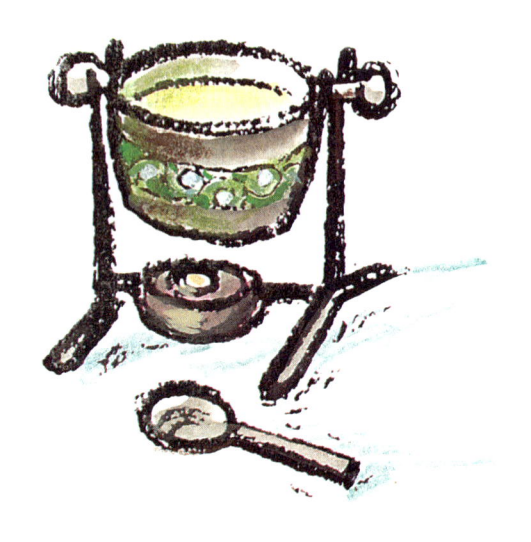

SPECIAL DIETS

Calories per SV	Protein g/ SV	Full-Liquid	Soft	Fiber-Restricted	Low-Lactose
90	1			*	

* Count as 1 serving of fruit out of daily allowance.

This is an old standby that is still popular. Serve it hot or chilled.

Rice Pudding

1 tbsp. cornstarch
1 1/2 tbsp. granulated sugar
1 beaten egg

1 cup milk
1/2 cup well cooked rice
1/2 tsp. vanilla

Blend first three ingredients in saucepan until smooth. Add milk slowly, stirring to mix well. Add rice. Cook over medium heat, stirring constantly until mixture is thickened and comes to a boil. Remove from heat, add vanilla, and cool. Sprinkle with cinnamon and nutmeg if desired. Many prefer rice pudding served warm. Try it for a new taste treat. Serves 3.

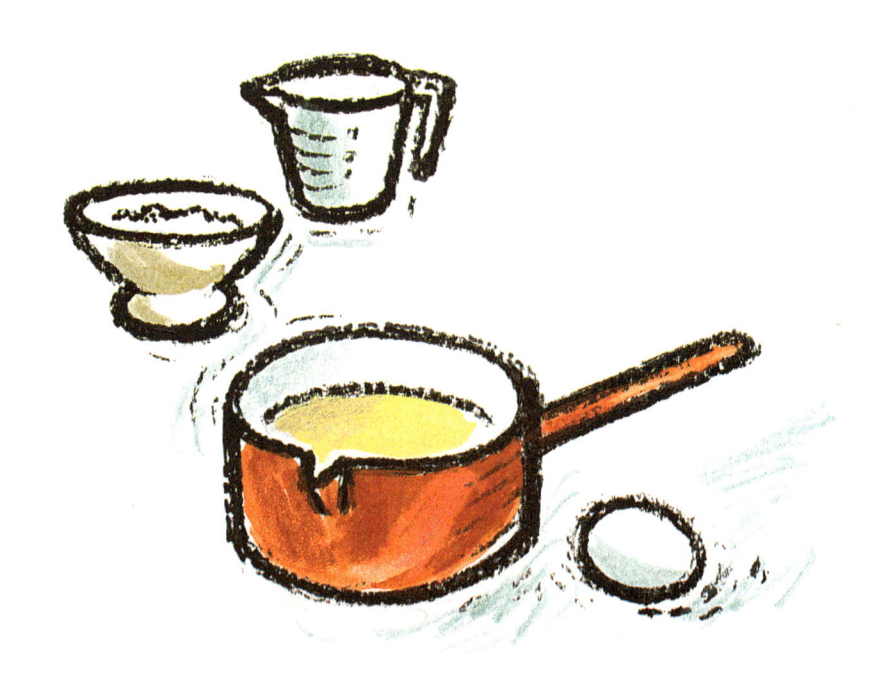

SPECIAL DIETS

Calories per SV	Protein g/ SV	Full-Liquid	Soft	Fiber-Restricted	Low-Lactose
140	6			**	*

* Substitute soy formula for milk.
** Each serving counts as 1/3 cup of milk.

Chocolate dessert lovers take note.

Milk-Free Double Chocolate Pudding

2 squares baking chocolate (1 oz. each)
1 tbsp. cornstarch
1/4 cup granulated sugar
1 cup nondairy creamer or soy formula
1 tsp. vanilla

Melt chocolate in small pan or on foil. Measure cornstarch and sugar into saucepan. Add part of the creamer and stir until cornstarch dissolves. Add the remainder of the creamer. Cook over medium heat until warm. Stir in chocolate until mixture is thick and comes to a boil. Remove from heat. Blend in vanilla and cool. Serves 2.

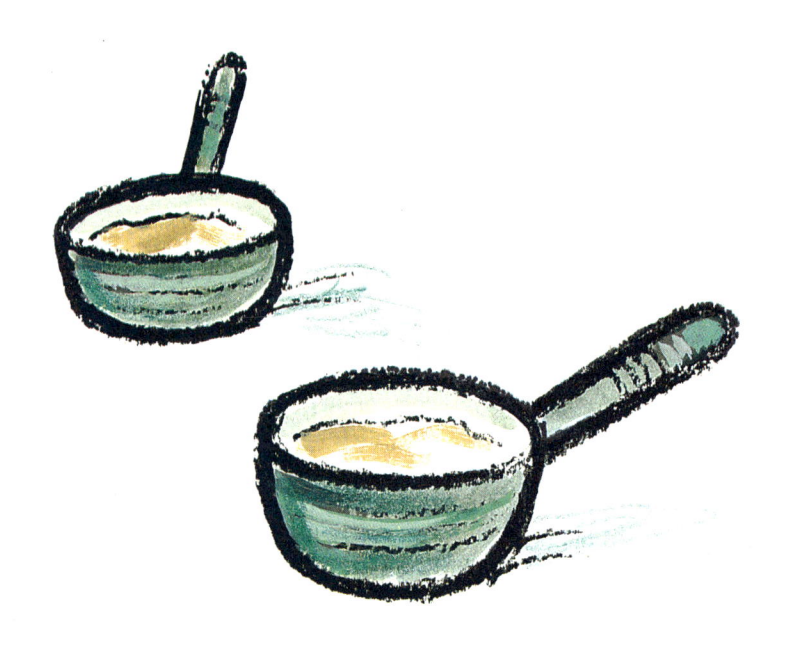

SPECIAL DIETS

Calories per SV	Protein g/ SV	Full-Liquid	Soft	Fiber-Restricted	Low-Lactose

WITH SOY FORMULA

370	11				

WITH NONDAIRY CREAMER

455	5				

Here is a pleasant dessert for those with a "sweet tooth" who cannot drink milk.

Milk-Free Vanilla Pudding

¼ cup sugar
2 tbsp. cornstarch
2 cups soy protein formula

1 egg, beaten
1 tsp. vanilla

Measure sugar and cornstarch into saucepan. Add a little of the soy formula. Stir to dissolve cornstarch, then pour in the rest of the liquid. Add beaten egg. Cook over medium heat until it comes to a boil and is thickened. Add vanilla and cool. Serves 4.

Maple Pudding: Omit vanilla and add ½ tsp. maple flavoring.

Maple-Nut Pudding: Add ¼ to ½ cup chopped walnuts or pecans to cooled pudding (not permitted on soft diet).

Coconut Pudding: Add ¼ cup coconut. Read the ingredient listing on coconut to be sure it has no lactose added (not permitted on soft diet).

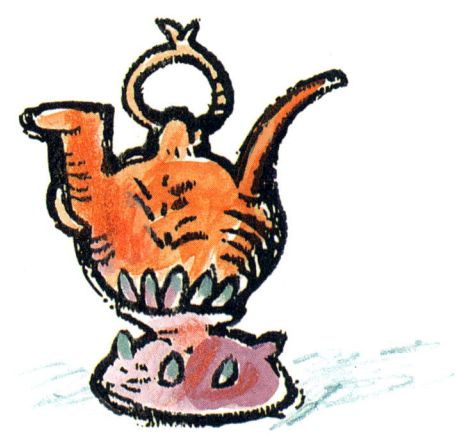

SPECIAL DIETS

	Calories per SV	Protein g/ SV	Full-Liquid	Soft	Fiber-Restricted	Low-Lactose
VANILLA/MAPLE	159	4				
MAPLE-NUT	207-255	5-6				
COCONUT	218	4				

Imitation ice cream— it's delightful and delicious.

Super Frozen Delight

1 package instant pudding (chocolate, vanilla, butterscotch, or lemon)

2 cups of chilled soy protein formula
2 cups nondairy whipped topping

Read the label of pudding mix to see that no milk or other milk product has been included. Prepare pudding as directed, substituting soy protein formula for milk. Gently fold in whipped topping. Pour into freezer container, cover, and freeze until firm, about 3 hours. Makes 1 quart. Serves 8.

Nut Delight: Fold in 1 cup of your favorite chopped nuts with the whipped topping *(not permitted on soft diet)*.

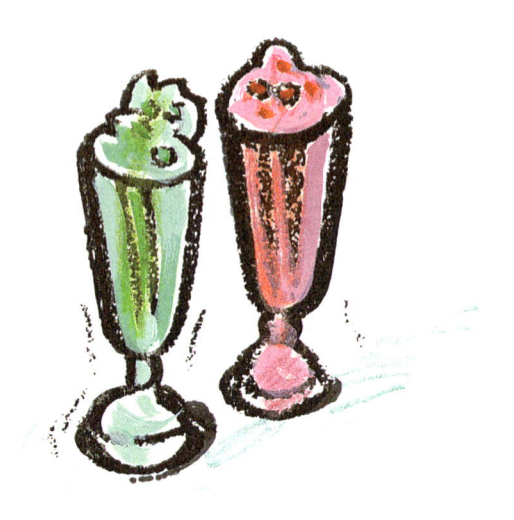

Calories per SV	Protein g/ SV	Full-Liquid	Soft	Fiber-Restricted	Low-Lactose
133	1				

SPECIAL DIETS

Recipe Index

Adair's Apple Raisin Cake   82
Amaretto Creme   75
Apple Brown Betty   81
Apple Cheese Betty   81
Apple Raisin Cake, Adair's   82
Banana-Butterscotch Milkshake   71
Banana Milkshake, Vera's   68
Banana-Nut Bread   84
Basic Meatloaf or Meatballs   54
Butterscotch-Banana Fake Shake   71
Butterscotch Brandy Creme   75
Butterscotch Fake Shake   71

Casseroles
   Robert's Tuna Bake   59
   Tuna Broccoli   60

Cheese Pies, Individual   81
Cheese-Spinach Pie   53
Cheesy Hamburger Casserole   52
Chicken Noodle Bake   58
Chicken Skillet Supper   58
Chicken Supreme   57
Chocolate Chip Granola   79
Chocolate Fake Shake   71
Citrus Fake Shakes   71
Coconut Pudding   91
Cowboy Cookies   86
Creamy Chicken Skillet Supper   58
Creamy Potato Salad   61
Creme de Menthe Smoothie   74
Creole Sauce   62
Double Chocolate Pudding, Milk-Free   90

Drinks With Alcohol
   Amaretto Creme   75
   Butterscotch Brandy Creme   75
   Creme de Menthe Smoothie   74
   Fruit Smoothie   74
   Panamanian   74

Fake Shake Sherbet   72

Fake Shakes
   Butterscotch   71
   Butterscotch-Banana   71
   Chocolate   71
   Citrus   71
   Peanut Butter-Honey   71

Fluffy Fruit Gelatin   88
Fortified Milk   67
Fresh Peach Sauce   76
Frosting, Helen's Soft Chocolate   85

Frozen Delight
   Super   92
   Nut   92
Frozen Fake Shakes   72

Fruit Smoothie   74

Granola
   Bars   80
   Chocolate Chip   79
   Granola I   79
   Granola II   79
   Raisin   79

Hamburger
   Sloppy Joes   55
   Cheesy Hamburger Casserole   52

Helen's Soft Chocolate Frosting   85
High-Protein Milkshakes   70
High-Protein Pancakes   65
Homemade Peanut Butter Shake   72

Individual Cheese Pies   83

Instant Breakfast Shake   72

Low-Lactose Pancakes   66
Macaroni and Cheese   51
Make-Your-Own Shake   72
Maple Nut Pudding   91
Maple Pudding   91

Meatballs
   Basic   54
   Swedish   56

Meatloaf, Basic   54

Milk
   Fortified   67
   Milk-Free Butterscotch Sauce   77
   Milk-Free Chocolate Sauce   71
   Milk-Free Double Chocolate Pudding   90
   Milk-Free Vanilla Pudding   91

Milkshakes
   Banana   68
   Banana Butterscotch   68
   Butterscotch Banana Fake Shake   71
   Butterscotch Fake Shake   71
   Chocolate Fake Shake   71
   Citrus Fake Shakes   71
   High-Protein   70
   Peanut Butter-Honey Fake Shake   71
   Strawberry, Pearl's   69

Molasses Taffy Snack Spread   78
Nut Frozen Delight   92

Pancakes
   Low-Lactose   66
   High-Protein   65

Panamanian Smoothie   74
Peanut Butter Bars   87
Peanut Butter-Honey Fake Shake   71
Peanut Butter Snack Spread   78

Pearl's Strawberry Milkshake   69

Potato Salad
   Creamy   61
   Ricotta   61

Puddings
   Coconut   91
   Maple   91
   Maple Nut   91
   Milk-Free Double Chocolate   90
   Milk-Free Vanilla   91
   Nut Frozen Delight   92
   Rice   89
   Super Frozen Delight   92

Quick Barbecue Sauce   63
Raisin Granola   79
Rice Pudding   89
Ricotta Potato Salad   61
Robert's Tuna Bake   59

Sauces
   Butterscotch, Milk-Free   77
   Chocolate, Milk-Free   71
   Creole   62
   Free Peach   76
   Milk-Free Butterscotch   77
   Quick Barbecue   63
   Sweet and Sour   64

Sloppy Joes   55
Strawberry Milkshake, Pearl's   69
Super Frozen Delight   92
Swedish Meatballs   56
Sweet and Sour Sauce   64
Tomato Chicken Skillet Supper   58
Tuna Bake, Robert's   59
Tuna Broccoli Casserole   60
Vanilla Pudding, Milk-Free   91
Vera's Banana Milkshake   68